Extrovert

Introvert Power to Live Like an Extrovert

(Unlock the Next Level of Yourself to Reap Incredible Benefits)

Victoria Rutland

Published By **Bengion Cosalas**

Victoria Rutland

All Rights Reserved

Extrovert: Introvert Power to Live Like an Extrovert (Unlock the Next Level of Yourself to Reap Incredible Benefits)

ISBN   978-1-77485-977-3

No part of this guidebook shall be reproduced in any form without permission in writing from the publisher except in the case of brief quotations embodied in critical articles or reviews.

Legal & Disclaimer

The information contained in this ebook is not designed to replace or take the place of any form of medicine or professional medical advice. The information in this ebook has been provided for educational & entertainment purposes only.

The information contained in this book has been compiled from sources deemed reliable, and it is accurate to the best of the Author's knowledge; however, the Author cannot guarantee its accuracy and validity and cannot be held liable for any errors or omissions. Changes are periodically made to this book. You must consult your doctor or get professional medical advice before using any of the suggested remedies, techniques, or information in this book.

Upon using the information contained in this book, you agree to hold harmless the Author from and against any damages, costs, and expenses, including any legal fees potentially resulting from the application of any of the information provided by this guide. This disclaimer applies to any damages or injury caused by the use and application, whether directly or indirectly, of any advice or information presented, whether for breach of contract, tort, negligence, personal injury, criminal intent, or under any other cause of action.

You agree to accept all risks of using the information presented inside this book. You need to consult a professional medical practitioner in order to ensure you are both able and healthy enough to participate in this program.

TABLE OF CONTENTS

Chapter 1: is about Introversion And Its Different Types

Introversion is one of the terms that is misinterpreted by the majority of us and people consider it to be shyness, but the truth is that there is no negative behavior among introverts. Their minds are actually created in a different way by their nature and is programmed to operate in a particular way, and everyone who is an introvert needs to recognize that while they face some limitations however, they also have certain benefits.

You've probably read about introverts many times, and you've were taught about their distinct characteristics from extroverts. But did you think all introverts can be classified in certain categories based on certain differences in their personality traits? It's true that the way introverts behave in social situations could differ from that of an extrovert in the same setting.

The research has shown it is possible to identify four types of introverts , based on the degree of this trait within them. They are as follows:

1.) Thinking Introverts

2.) Social Introverts

3.) Restrained Introverts

4.) Anxious Introverts

Let's look at these introversions in order you'll be able to figure out which type of introversion you are faced with.

Thinking Introverts

There are some introverts that prefer to sit quietly and pondering anything that happens around them or has that has happened to them recently within the last few years. They are naturally drawn to being worried about the things they see around them. They can easily become worried about small things and continue to think about them until they can return to normal.

If introverts who think are asked to analyze something it is easy for them to accomplish this and possibly better than extroverts since their character traits give them the ability to evaluate every detail, event or other event that is important.

Social Introverts

Social introverts like to be in their own space and like it when nobody is around and they are able to spend their time doing the things they love to do. They try to stay away from socializing whenever they can, and if they have to do so in certain situations the majority of them stay with a few friends or within a group that they are already a part of.

Social introverts feel exhausted to a large extent in social settings and are eagerly waiting to get into silence to recuperate and regain their normal energy levels. The presence of so many people drains their minds and emotions, and even their bodies and they are in desperate need of to find a way out.

People who have this kind of introversion are often regarded as shy, but there is no evidence similar to that. If you're an introverted social person it doesn't suggest that there is a lack of confidence within your character and that you're scared of the world. It's just that you're someone with a distinct mind that is different from the minds of those whom you usually meet in a social circle.

Restricted Introverts

These types of introverts are rare. They are the ones who need an amount of time to become accustomed to new situations. Once they have, they are capable of engaging in fascinating conversations with other people and winning their hearts. The people who exhibit this type of introversion are referred to as restrained introverts. they enjoy attending an event they've been to a couple of times in the past and are a part of it as every other extrovert.

A common trait among introverts of this kind is that they tend to think about their thoughts before speaking in any setting and this is their strength.

Anxious Introverts

According to the title, introverts who feel anxious when in a crowd are referred to as anxious introverts. These kinds of introverts aren't as comfortable being on their own in the same way that people with other types , but their presence in a social setting causes them to feel anxious and they begin to experience awkward emotions. In the end, they'd like to get out of the area as soon as they can.

The behaviors of people who have the type of personality might be related to instances or social interactions that occurred during the last few years. The anxious introverts require more time and attention than other kind of introvert because they have a very tender heart and are prone to getting injured easily by small things. These people require proper guidance to help them deal anxiety and gain confidence in their social lives that will help them achieve success in their lives.

Whatever type of introversion that you encounter, you must be aware that it isn't an issue or weakness however it is a form of personality you possess. Instead of focusing on it as an obstacle to your path of success, consider how you can make use of it to help you advance in your career because there's always something unique that God has gifted everyone with It's just a problem of being aware of it.

Introverted Qualities

Many introverts are viewed as anxious socially, but this is not the case. It is possible that you are hesitant to engage with others in certain social settings but it doesn't suggest that you're afraid of people when you are in large groups.

An introvert is able to dominate any setting and handle difficult conversations the same way that extroverts do It's a issue of recognizing the strengths and applying them in the correct way.

In this section, you'll discover some of the most well-known qualities you could have as an introvert but may not be aware of them.

Introverts Can Find Happiness Easily

If you're an introvert, you'll effortlessly find happiness doing something at home you love the most, such as watching your favorite TV show on the television or reading a great book unlike extroverts who must invest money in their enjoyment, such as having a night out with friends, as well as paying for travel expenses and expensive meals. Therefore, it's simple for introverts to get some satisfaction and be more content than extroverts.

Introverts are observant.

The ability of introverts to observe is extremely sharp as they quickly detect changes happening to their environment. If someone experienced changes in their internal environment or body, or someone was healthier or less so than the last time they were there or saw a face that was similar with someone else They would be able to immediately recognize the changes.

Most of the time the power of this kind of analysis is appreciated by other as they are unable to be aware of such changes , but you make them aware of the changes.

Introverts are trustworthy

It is a factor that can make your connections with your friends and family members lasting and doesn't let them fall apart when tough times occur.

Introverts can be trusted with keeping secrets as they are aware of the importance of being reliable. They will never divulge any personal information about people they have good terms with and this shows they're better friends than the rest of us.

Introverts are goal-oriented

Goal-oriented individuals are an important citizens of society who are determined to achieve something greater in their lives. This will not only benefit them , but also those who surround them.

Introverts are those who define the goals they want to achieve and strive to achieve success in their chosen field.

People who are introverts can be good listeners.

Introverts are capable to listen better than extroverts , and they won't join any conversation without listening to everything with attention and know the significance of the conversation. They are prepared before speaking before anyone else, and this makes people speak with confidence.

You will benefit by this skill as an introvert and make use of your listening skills in a variety of social settings to protect your self from awkward situations when you are unsure of how to speak or how to react to people who are asking questions about a specific issue in the event of not having adequate listening skills.

Introverts aren't averse to relying on others

Introverts tend to be being able to do everything by themselves, without being dependent on others. They don't rely on others to be there for them confronted with a problem and try to deal any challenge on their own.

This gives them the confidence that they will be able to face any challenge in life and get through it successfully. This is why introverts are not scared of facing the biggest challenges of life.

Introverts have Great Focus

We all know that the success of any project and to achieve higher results than expected is something that requires more focus and attention. The introverts are able to stay completely focused on the task at hand or even becoming part of.

This skill helps them to comprehend all things properly, and helps prevent them from making errors.

People who are introverts Fond of Study

It's true that every person who is interested in learning and is always eager to know more about things is more likely to achieve being successful over those who show less curiosity about learning.

Introverts enjoy learning and particularly of acquiring new skills that will help them be successful in their fields. This habit provides them with ability to learn as they age and they are a valuable benefit to society.

Introverts can control their feelings

Introverts are well-aware of how to handle their emotions since they know that they are emotional.

This skill helps to keep their emotions in check when confronted with situations that can hurt their feelings, which can make them feel unhappy, angry, guilty or anxious. They are able to easily overcome negative thoughts in their mind and remain cool in front of others.

Introverts like to discuss the most important things only

The truth is that introverts do not like conversations like extroverts, but that doesn't suggest that they aren't capable of having an engaging conversation, and conversing in a way that is interesting.

What's different about introverts is that they aren't averse to having conversations or discussing topics that aren't important to them, however they can be able to discuss any important subject that is important to them from their own way as well like any other individual do.

Introverted Characteristics

If you prefer spending relaxing at home and with family or with friends instead of going out to social gatherings You are probably an introvert. You have certain traits that distinguish you from the other people who are extroverts.

There is a common belief that introverts do not like public speaking because they don't feel at ease in public settings and would prefer to get away from crowds. In reality, introverts are competent at speaking to a crowd and deliver a memorable speech if they're well-prepared for the task and the topic is of passion.

There are numerous influential individuals and self-made businessmen around the world who have achieved success throughout their lives despite their being introverts. This shows that introversion is not a problem that stands in the way of your success If you're looking to make a difference for yourself, the only thing you require is determination and determination.

There is no doubt that the way an introvert behaves in certain situations may differ from one another, however there are certain traits that can be found in every introvert. In this article, we'll look at some of the most prevalent traits that introverts share and how they can help you to succeed in life as an introvert.

Introverts don't like Small Talk

People who are introverted do not like small talk because they feel like they are tired, while extroverts feel more energetic as they spend more time on small talk.

It doesn't mean introverts aren't able to create a successful conversation like extroverts. The issue is that they prefer to speak about things that matter or concepts.

Introverts Should Avoid Crowds

People who are introverts don't like crowds like when they're in a social setting and are always waiting to find a private space where they can be alone.

If they're alone they are able to think and comprehend more clearly what is happening in the present, which can help them feel more relaxed.

Introverts Love Going for walks

One very healthy and beneficial habit introverts develop is that they like long walks in the early morning or late in the evening. They are attracted to the objects around them since they naturally tend to be absorbed by anything that happens to them or encounter.

They enjoy going to parks or gardens because they are attracted by the greenery, and also they would like to take a break free from the stresses of their daily lives that leave them exhausted and tired.

Introverts are able to hide their emotions

There are times when people struggle to control their emotions. They are unable to express their feelings even in inappropriate settings and this can lead to embarrassments both for themselves and for those around them.

Introverts have the capacity to conceal their emotions and feelings whenever they'd like, and they can avoid making scenes in a variety of circumstances where they feel very angry or sad.

Introverts make few friends.

Introverts are extremely selective in how they selecting their friends since they are not averse to having more than they need. Many people believe that introverts are shy . However, in reality, they prefer to be able to spend some time in solitude , where they are able to think and think about the most important moments in their lives and take crucial choices.

They require time for themselves to develop their lives as they are goal-oriented individuals which is why they aren't able to meet new people and form friendships after observing with just a few individuals in their social circle that share a likeness to their ideas and opinions.

Introverts hate Limelight

They don't have the need of being in the limelight every day as extroverts do. They are keen to have people interested in their activities and strive to attract attention from everyone.

Introverts prefer to do their work in silence without announcements or boasting about the things they have achieved or are able to be able to achieve.

Introverts aren't interested in talking about Theyself

Introverts aren't keen on talking about themselves, but like to hear from others rather. They don't feel confident about talking about their dislikes, likes and thoughts on particular subjects or expressing what they are doing in their daily lives. They don't want to appear proud or let people believe that they're proud of something that they've done.

This doesn't mean introverts aren't honest about themselves . They hide all things that are related to them, but they do share their personal information with those they are able to trust.

Introverts can recognize strengths of others

When you have to judge others and giving them the right direction to progress in their field Introverts are always there to assist.

They monitor each member of the team and communicate to them what they're lacking by reviewing your strengths and weakness. This is why they have leadership qualities that they can apply in their business and be successful entrepreneurs.

Introverts can work in a team

Introverts don't like being dependent on other people and prefer to complete the work by themselves.

They are an invaluable member of a team because they are able to produce impressive results thanks to their determination and commitment.

The reason for this is that they possess the ability to work with enthusiasm and produce amazing accomplishments in their professional lives.

Introverts aren't the only ones who don't speak first.

Extroverts are known to like having their voice heard or to make announcements but introverts might not be the first to speak at any gathering because of their inherent hesitation.

Extroverts are at ease attracting the attention of many people, and that's why they can talk anywhere they want with no one's help. What introverts have in common is that they would like being accompanied by someone when speaking to the crowd or at any gathering as it helps them feel at ease and they are able to easily communicate with people of all ages.

Introverts like to spend time at home, mostly

The introverts aren't interested in attending numerous social or party occasions every weekend, however, they prefer to relax at home and watch their favourite film or show.

However, this doesn't mean they don't value their buddies, but they desire to stay in touch with their buddies and enjoy fun with their friends from time to time. They just want some space and a quiet space where no one disturbs them, not even their friends.

People who are introverts want to stay away from the phone

Focus is is essential when doing important tasks. Introverts are those who are extremely focused and don't like any interruption.

When they're doing something that is crucial, they will not let anyone to interrupt them, not even a telephone calls. They are of the opinion that directing their attention to someone else or answering the phone would cause them to lose their momentum, which was not created by them. This is why they do not leave the work for another thing until they've completed it completely or even a small portion of it.

Introverts are creative

Nearly in every industry, there is a demand for innovative people with unique concepts for the expansion and growth of the company.

Introverts are creative because they are able of thinking in a unique manner and often create valuable ideas that are appreciated by all.

They don't worry about what other people think of them but they keep up their work with a lot of effort and commitment, and finally achieve amazing results using their imaginative minds.

Chapter 2: The Best Ways to Make Small Talk
The art of making small talk is challenging for those who are introvert. However, it is simpler if you employ specific strategies. Everyone would like to be appreciated for their interactions with other people at social gatherings, however very few are able to impress other people by their manner of speaking.

This chapter will concentrate on techniques you can use to have a successful small conversation with people you meet in your daily day life, as an introvert, and make them feel loved.

Pay attention to what others Say

If you pretend to participate in conversations and do not pay attention to the opinions of others they'll think that you don't care about what they might say to you. This could cause others to think that they're being disrespected and that things could happen similar to what they see from their perspective. This means that the small discussion could be disrupted.

To avoid this circumstance, it is important to demonstrate some genuineness to your fellows and respect their opinions. You don't have to show your attentiveness when you utilize your capacity to listen to fully comprehend the message from the opposite side.

Be Confident

Learn to be a good judge of others for what they are good at in their lives. When you express your admiration for them you feel happy and want to reciprocate similarly.

If you are interested in other people, you improve the likelihood of being liked also, since you display your confidence in by doing this. It's been proven that, of all traits confident is one of the ones that make you attractive to people.

Keep a smile on your face and keep smiling

It's not required to be happy constantly as there are many issues happening in our lives every day and we might be unhappy too when we need to have small-sized talk with somebody.

If you maintain a smile on your face and strive to appear happy even although you might not appear so at all times, you will enhance the enjoyment of your conversation and the person you're communicating with will be feeling much more comfortable.

Remember the good times you've recently experienced: Enjoyment at a weekend's gathering, having laughter with your friends or any other incident that brought you to laughter. Your smile that is happy can help create a the right atmosphere.

Connect Your Conversation to Previous One

One of the most effective strategies for making a smart small talk is to follow up on information that you learn from other people in the conversation. You could ask them a question about something connected to the topic they're discussing and then give them the chance to explain and provide you with additional information to give your opinions on.

Utilizing this tactic in conversation can save you a lots of time and energy when making efforts to find something fresh to say at the end of the conversation.

Use Perfume

The scent of a light perfume can help you feel more comfortable as an introverted individual. It has been proven that those who wear mild lemon-scented scent improve their confidence when going to a public event.

Your appearance is attractive and can make people feel happy everywhere you go.

Have a friendly attitude

One of the issues introverts encounter in conversation is showing interest in other people. It is vital to establish relationships, particularly with colleagues or neighbors at work.

If you're speaking to someone you've had an interactions with in the time, you could discuss any event that was part of the conversation that took place at the time , or something interesting discussed, such as the weekend plans, launching an enterprise or buying a new car , etc. It will allow you to demonstrate your enthusiasm for others in this manner and will also help you feel more comfortable speaking to them.

Write about your experiences

Be mindful of what can put the conversation off the right track , and what stops it eventually and that is usually speaking negatively about someone else, like the backbiting or blaming. This isn't a good thing to do, and it reduces your popularity in the eyes of others. The more positive you speak about yourself, the more enjoyable the discussion will turn out to be.

You could share some memorable memories from your past or make a humorous joke that will make people laugh , since this method is thought to be the most effective in being appreciated by everyone.

Try to be humble

There are people who attempt to conceal their flaws and appear flawless in front of everyone however this method doesn't work.

The psychology of psychology has shown that people because they are willing to share their shortcomings or the mistakes they make in their daily lives as opposed to those who are afraid to tell others about the wrongs they committed.

Making mistakes is not just a matter of self-reflection but also will make you look more confident, humble, and frees you from any guilt and makes people believe that you're not a hypocrite , but an ordinary human being just as they are.

Improve Social Skills

Social skills play an essential part in achieving success both in your professional and personal lives. If you master the art of connecting with others and establishing solid relationships, you is always at hand.

The majority of introverted women don't make a negative impression on other people because their weaknesses as introverts are hidden by their egoism or timidity in the eyes of others, especially when they are beautiful. But , people view things differently with regards to the men's social skills. They need to improve their social skills by taking every step towards becoming a confident social person.

Know Your Strengths as a Gender

Men who are introverted can make an impression that is positive, just as women who are more introverted can, however they must approach things differently. We have already seen how women strive to present themselves as attractive when they're lacking in social abilities.

Men can strive to be as relaxed as they can and build self-confidence that can help people view their character from a positive angle.

Choose Carefully What to Wear

You can make an excellent impression by your choice of clothing by keeping up with the latest trends in fashion that are popular with people, particularly when you believe that you won't be able to grab the attention of everyone with your choice of speaking.

You'll also feel more relaxed and secure in your abilities and eventually you will be able to be able to see people engaging with you on their own because they naturally will be attracted to you.

Talk when it is necessary

Don't think you must be too loud, especially when you're part of the conversation with the company of strangers. Since you're a new person to them, they may not be familiar with your character or opinions regarding the things that they are most interested in. They don't also think you'll be able to speak many things about their beliefs or interests since you haven't interacted with them previously, and therefore, you don't have any idea about their beliefs.

Be calm and pay attention to the conversation fully and speak up with confidence, if you believe it's necessary to say it without worrying about the way everyone reacts to it.

Learn the Ways to Communicate

If you're participant at a social gathering in which people are familiar with you and you know many or all of them, something you should be careful about is to listen thoroughly, take in their thoughts, and consider what you need to say, and then respond with the correct manner.

The issue of introverts lies in the fact that they are able to think and listen onlyand don't react in the same way. On the other hand, extroverts respond and listen They don't think about what they're supposed to say and then they express their opinion instantly.

Talk in a friendly Way

Conversation with strangers as strangers is something many of us do, but it is not a good method to build connections. Send them a warm and welcoming greeting as well as make them feel that you've known them for long. Because nobody wants to speak to people who make them feel as if they are a stranger.

The more positive tone you employ with them, the greater chance of strong bonds you establish with them. This is the art of quickly making friends and retaining their hearts with a loving and friendly manner of speaking.

Be aware of the latest trends in fashion.

Be aware of the recent topics people love to discuss, and then practice speaking about them, regardless of whether you're alone or with someone else. You can build your confidence slowly.

Extroverts have the ability of engaging in conversation about the latest trends because they're confident and also perform it regularly. When you are able to maintain regularity to your interactions with other people on topics like that, you're just a few steps away from mastering this skill.

You don't need to be a Witty person.

The truth is that engaging other people is a talent that is not widely understood. There are those who quickly attract the attention of the crowd with their unique style of talking and also entertain them , however there are people who aren't able to succeed.

They are unique and aren't comfortable at the center of attention. If you're into this category, you shouldn't have to be concerned about anything There is no way to make you do anything you're not comfortable with.

Don't be a lone wolf, be member of the crowd for the duration of the conversation. This ensures that no one feels something odd about your presence.

Pick the Right Place to Meet strangers

The biggest issue introverts have has to do with the fact that it is difficult to initiate conversations when they meet one at first. Especially when meeting someone with a different sex It is likely that you'll be in this kind of circumstances.

A meeting with someone at an environment where you discover something exciting or novel to talk about, may be the answer to this issue since you can easily begin conversations. If you happen to be at a popular eatery, you can discuss about their food and appreciate it, or discuss their views.

In contrast, if you are inviting them to an open area there's nothing interesting to discuss and the conversation could end into a monotonous manner.

Spend some time enjoying

It's essential to recharge your brain by doing something that is enjoyable for you in addition to the stress of the day-to-day routine of the many things you do. Choose what you love the most during your free time. You can play any sport, watch the most popular movie or read a great book, or have a date for dinner or lunch with any of your closest acquaintances.

In this way, you'll be able free your mind to let new ideas flow, so that you'll have something fresh to discuss. Our confidence is in our heads and your main focus is on building confidence and increasing your social abilities.

Be serious and don't fret about what others consider about you and you've done in the entire process, because once you have achieved your goals, they will definitely appreciate you.

Be aware of your strengths

It is important to evaluate yourself and find out your strengths. You may be a skilled speaker, a good listener or possess a powerful body language. Whatever your skill it is important to make the most of it to ensure that people see your accomplishments with a wistful eye.

Chapter 3: Compete with Extroverts

Being an introvert can be difficult when it comes to going to social gatherings, social events or any public speaking event. If you're a sufferer of introversion is the biggest challenge you can face in these situations. In this article you will learn efficient tips you can use to get over this obstacle and make life simple for you.

If you live your life of an introvert, or are naturally that you're aware that success in the modern world is only for people who are extroverts. Things are much simpler for them, whether it's for them to excel in their professional lives or to build relationships in their private lives. They are quick to meet new friends and everyone is eager to be part of their group everywhere they go in the social group.

One of the most obvious characteristics of an introvert is to be invisible everywhere, whether at college as a pupil, the workplace as an employee or even at the party as guests. It is always a good idea to remain in a quiet corner after a some interaction with people dependent on your level of energy. You will try to find an area that is quiet because you are able to regain your energy only when you're alone.

Extroverts feel more energetic when in a crowd and like to engage in some sort of sport or enjoy themselves most times. They enjoy this the most . The more time they devote to this they gain more socially active they become. This allows people to express their thoughts and opinions easily and quickly.

It's also a proven fact that although no one is completely extrovert or introverted. However, if you look at the research There is a specific proportion of people who belong to one of the categories more than the other. You can conduct an analysis using these signs and determine what your introversion level is. Higher your level and the more concentration you'll have to pay attention to your safety in a world full of extroverts.

Don't let the thought persist within your mind that the universe is just for those who are extroverts and that people who are introverts can't achieve anything in their lives. This is a huge myth that a lot of people believe However, you have to be sure of yourself first, and concentrate on how you can achieve success both in your professional and personal life, where you must contend with a variety of extroverts.

Let's examine the tactics you have to follow for survival amid the sea of extroverts and be more successful as an introvert.

Create Everything on paper

The introverts have a higher likelihood communicate their thoughts and feelings in writing than speaking. Conversely, people who are extroverts have a natural ability to speak and are able to express their thoughts or feelings via verbal communication with ease.

Use this to your advantage and use it to write your thoughts on sheet prior to going to any social gathering or event. If you're attending an interview for a job You can note down the key points that you will be asked at the time of the interview. Check everything you write down on the paper a couple of times to ensure you've stated everything in a proper manner and that nothing is left out.

The purpose of this method is to aids you in navigating the conversation with no awkward pauses since you already have an order to your thoughts on paper and you have practiced the process of reading them in order to make them perfect in your head.

Find Info about the People You Meet

When you meet individuals who are new to you, it's important to get to know them in the best way you can. So, you'll be able to assess yourself to others and discover the similarities and differences observed between you in regards to your likes and dislikes, and other things.

Look up the profiles of their social media or any other online platform because it can help you learn more about their character and the type of person they might be.

For work-related or business meeting with people who are not your friends, follow the same procedure and plan well to ensure that your meeting is productive by avoiding awkward times of conversation. You can learn more regarding them through their LinkedIn profile. It will give you information on their professional skills and experiences.

You can also reach them via email or telephone and tell them some details about yourself and the the location that would be ideal to have a meeting for each of you.

Use Social Media

If you're not able to meet a similar person in your vicinity, you could utilize social media or an internet-based platform, where you'll encounter a variety of people, whose thinking of which matches your own. You can form online friendships with anyone you are interested in and meeting them will be enjoyable when you go into the crowd of extroverts at social gatherings.

Social events, parties or even a gathering of the family is a nightmare for introverts, and they want to escape as much as possible. Being an introvert doesn't necessarily mean you are shy or anxious, however introverts have strengths that the majority of people don't know about and they can prove they are helpful when fighting with extroverts.

An introvert is a superior listener than other people and this can enable them to communicate confidently. Focus on this quality and use it when needed to feel happy.

Introverts do not like spaces that are loud or filled with people however, they would like to gather in places with small interactions. They also enjoy going to places where they can meet people with similar thinking to their own. Therefore, it's beneficial for you, an introvert, to be in a location.

Be aware of your Qualities

While there are certain abilities introverts lack when it comes to making it in the world of extroverts, however, you shouldn't be worried because as an introvert you possess certain characteristics which give you an advantage over extroverts.

Each introvert has inborn capabilities that are superior to those who benefit from the advantages of the extrovert. Perhaps you're a great listener, extremely focused or extremely observant. What you have to do is to identify all these talents and work to improve them to the maximum extent you can and discover how to use these skills to your advantage.

Be selective in attending social Evenings

Extroverts wait eagerly for the day when they will be off work and get an opportunity to dine with their family or friends for dinner and enjoy a night out with their friends. For introverts, life is different because they don't wish to be around anyone when they return home, especially after a long and exhausting shift at work.

There is no requirement to attend every business or social gathering in the same way, but you are able to pick among them only those which are most important to you and cannot afford to miss these events. You must think from a the perspective of a realistic person when you accept invitations, rather than getting anxious or worrying what other people might consider if you didn't attend the event.

In your private life rather than committing yourself to the idea of hosting social gatherings at any time of the day or at night, choose the weekend as the best time to host them because you're mentally free during that time to be an integral part of the event and relish every moment with your loved ones and friends.

Select the Job that is Right for You

To have an effective career in the field it is essential to locate an occupation that will suit you best for an introvert because not all jobs are suitable for people of all types.

Many people make the error of trying to mold their personal style into a job that is suited to extroverts . They waste lots of time doing this. At some point, they realize they're not suited for the job and they should leave.

It's best to take your decision when you are beginning your career. You can choose the job that is most suitable to your personality . This will ensure that you are more likely to build a an enviable career in that.

jobs that require public talking, networking, or cold calls are not suitable for introverts, but you could quickly make it in the field where more concentration, studying and listening abilities are needed to work in a team.

Accept the fact that life isn't easy for those who are introverts and you'll encounter obstacles at different stages in both your professional and personal life.

Make yourself appear like an extrovert

There are occasions in your daily life that require you to cover up your introversion completely otherwise you might get in trouble later and will regret not doing it.

This is particularly true when you attend an event for business, and you have an important information or an idea that you want to share, and want to communicate the idea to all attendees, however, despite your overwhelming desire, you don't accomplish this. It means that you cannot share the thoughts that are in your head due to your shy personality.

It is possible to prevent this situation from occurring by doing everything to share your ideas or anything else you wish to discuss during the meeting. The only thing you have to do is behave like an extrovert, assuming that you're an extrovert.

What you're doing is actually creating the illusion of extrovert, even though you might have a hard time doing this at first, however, you are able to keep your training and, as you progress you'll begin to feel more comfortable and confident about what you're doing.

Seize the Chance

People who are introverts do not like being the focus of attention at all times as extroverts do, but at times it's essential for them to step outside their comfort zone and do to attract everyone's attention.

As an example, say you're sitting in the classroom, attending a business conference or other gathering in which you have an inquiry to make or an important point to discuss or something intriguing to share with everyone Don't pass up the chance to give yourself the opportunity to increase your worth from a different perspective not as you're not looking make everyone else notice you.

Make sure to share your thoughts in your voice in a loud way and ensure that everyone around you is paying focus. You might not be able of making your voice sound as powerful as the other people, however, you must remember that you need to beat others in all areas to progress and be successful.

If you can keep this thought in your head it will give you motivation to tackle any task you're reluctant to tackle as an introvert.

Learn the art of Public Speaking

There may be times where you're with extroverts in any situation and it's bound to deliver an address to all. In this situation you'll need to go beyond your the comfort zone, step out of the shadows and give your voice heard with all the enthusiasm.

Learning to speak in public for handling situations like these could help you. You can take a class to improve your abilities and this is a great way that will lead to success in all aspect of your life.

There are competitors everywhere in this day and age and can't avoid success by avoiding it. There is no reason to be concerned about, you can be just as successful as every person who is extrovert, the only thing you have to concentrate on your strengths. Look into what you excel at opposed to the rest of us and utilize it as a useful tool to help you.

Job Interview Tips and Techniques

The preparation for an interview that is successful will require you to know the tips and tricks as an introvert so that you can follow the route that will help you get the job you've always wanted. Interviews aren't easy for anyone , but introverts ought to approach them with more seriousness and be prepared for each step before going to the interview.

If you find yourself in front of people who are strangers to you and are asked to talk about your skills and experiences you've had and the reasons why they should employ the person you're talking to, you're likely to feel quite nervous because of your shy nature.

Here you will discover some helpful techniques that will make small talk and self-promotion easier during the interview.

Know the best way to present yourself

Write a short introduction to yourself in just a just a couple of lines. It is a essential for each interview. It is a crucial aspect of the interview, especially for introverts as you could be anxious when introducing yourself in the event that you're not prepared and things can go wrong way.

It is possible to describe your professional expertise as well as your strengths, and previous achievements you've had in your professional career. Remember that you must not say anything that creates you with a negative impression.

Get ready for Common Questions

There are certain types of types of questions that are typical during every interview. These are referred to as typical interview questions. If you are an introvert, you may be uneasy answering a question that you have did not have before and that could lead to an awkward moment during the conversation.

To prevent this from happening, make an outline of the most basic questions you are likely to be asked during interviews. Then, practice answering them one-by-one while in front of the mirror.

If you're unsure regarding a particular question or is posed then you can get advice from any of your close friends or family members who have already gone through the same issue. The more you practice, the more proficient you'll be.

Learn to handle small Talk

As an introvert , you're not great in small talk and this can cause difficulties for you when are interviewed. Before you begin to introduce your own or even after, the interviewers might begin a conversation with you, and you need be prepared for it.

They could ask you something in addition to the standard interview questions, or discuss an experience with you to gain your perspective to determine your opinion about certain issues.

Make sure you are prepared to manage a small talk during the moment of interview. you'll be prepared with a few sentences you could use to describe the gorgeous weather or about anything that is good about the surrounding.

Do not forget that you're in the market for to get this job. You have to impress interviewers through establishing relationships with them.

You should dedicate your complete Energy to the interview

Many people make the error of scheduling several interviews in one day, and as a result their energy and focus is split.

There is a chance to be in big trouble If you do this since you're an introvert characteristic and meeting many people at once will cause you to be exhausted and tired and there is a chance that you will lose your job at a top business due to being unable to focus to go through that particular interview.

To be successful, it is important to concentrate on just one interview instead of making a lot of preparations in your the back of your mind. It is best to focus all your time and effort on just one company and only one interview one at a time.

This doesn't mean taking another interview the same day isn't a good decision, but it is all dependent on how you feel and if you think you are able to go through another interview giving the same enthusiasm then you should take it or else it might be unnecessary.

Remember Your Successes

They do have some characteristics which are essential to various organizations. They could prove to be a benefit to them by using all of those traits as their strengths.

If they are required to give an presentation or talk about things with their managers introverts don't have the confidence as others, but when it comes to their creativity or working on original concepts or undertakings that require attention to detail, it's introverts who are most effective.

Take a moment to think about all the exceptional actions you performed during your professional career and then write them down on paper. Try to imagine that through your introverted personality, you were able to do something more than other people. It could be a challenging task you had to complete or a complex job you accomplished before the deadline.

Keep Concentrated

Introverts are prone to lose their focus when they're at new locations and face strangers. They begin thinking about what is happening around them. It doesn't matter if it's a phone call or a picture hanging on the wall or a book lying placed on the table, do not allow your attention to wander away from the conversation.

Remember that those few minutes are crucial to your career , and may turn out to be a pivotal factor in your career success. Be attentive to what your an interviewer has to say or ask and then respond by paying attention to it.

Find Information on the Company

Find out all you possibly can on the business that you are scheduled to meet with during the interview. Visit their website for the most up-to-date information and news accessible on the internet. You have a clear idea of the job you've applied for, however it is crucial to know exactly what you'll be working on and what kinds of products or services are provided by the business.

This can give you an idea how well-known this company and how worthwhile working there could prove to be. The information you gain can also help you answer questions during the interview, especially if you are asked the information you have about the company.

If you are in contact with one among the companies, it is possible to get information from them, such as who from what positions are on the interview panel and also what you can expect from them in the interview.

It's great if can determine what time the conversation lasts for every candidate since it will assist you in preparing to be prepared.

Be Prepared for Unexpected Questions

Sometimes an interviewer asks questions that the interviewee isn't expecting , and the person is left wondering what to answer. This is when stalling strategies can be effective if you are more aware and know how to apply them correctly.

Be prepared for the situations ahead of time by learning the art of slowing down. You can prolong your time to comment on the question with the words "Great" and "Interesting" and then putting the smile to your face.

This creates an impression to interviewers that it was a pleasure to answer the interview question and that you have the ability to keep their attention away from getting an accurate answer but the reality is that you aren't able to avoid the question, and you need to respond.

Make a substitute response to your own mind as fast as you can about your capabilities and then try to demonstrate that you're doing something more than what they were looking for.

This is the best method to deal with the circumstance, rather than just telling them that you don't have an idea what they are talking about.

Don't let negative thoughts strike Your Mind

Maintaining a positive attitude during the interview is extremely crucial because If negative thoughts come into the mind of your interviewee, these may ruin your confidence and as a consequently your body language may be affected.

Interviewers don't just listen to what you say out loud, but they also pay close attention to the movements in your physique. They'll immediately realize that you've got a bit of fears in you and this may make them reduce your score.

A good way to combat with negative thoughts and thoughts is to tell yourself that this isn't the only company that you can perform the task in and there are many opportunities available to those who fail to land a job. This will help you gain an inner strength and courage to tackle any difficult situation that you encounter in the course of your interview.

Every company is not able to have everyone who is flawless, however there are strengths and weaknesses in each employee.

Your introversion is a your strength, it is a question of knowing you are an introvert. you and what talents do you have to be able to compete with the extroverts. Be confident in yourself and believe that you are a unique professional with specific capabilities.

New Employment Probable Obstacles

A new job can be a thrilling experience for someone looking to master new skills, but it can be stressful and nerve-wracking at same time for people who are introverts.

If you are planning to begin your new job, you'll certainly encounter challenges because you are an introvert. There will be many obstacles on your path. This section will focus on the most typical ones you're most likely to encounter in the new workplace.

Make Your Introduction

They don't like being at the centre of attention, as extroverts, and this hinders them from engaging within larger crowds.

Make a plan for the way you'll introduce yourself before everyone on your first day at the new job. You'll be more comfortable during the process if you prepare all the things you need to convey about you in your introduction.

You could write your points on the paper that pertain to your academic qualifications, your employment history, and any information regarding your hobbies, like what you do during your free time, etc.

Be able to say "No"

Examine things in the current environment to determine what you like and what isn't since there may be tasks you're offered in addition to your job that don't fit with your personal style.

Learn to decline those offers but at same time, don't be reluctant to accept those that you think would work best with your style.

It's a aspect of being willing to say no or yes to anything you're given. If you're asked to any kind of social gathering take part in it if you believe you are comfortable with the event, but don't be afraid to turn it down if you think the event unsuitable for your needs.

Be Specific About Your Work Style

Every person is different in their approach to working, but it's not required to be able to be liked or rejected by all. Although some people appreciate your approach to work but at the same time, there could be some who don't like your work style.

Being an introvert can confront this challenge, but you need to remain assured and you don't requirement to change how you work. The key to success is to recognize your strengths and trust them to show everyone by hard work, dedication and commitment that you're capable of accomplishing everything everyone in the company can.

Take A Break

The constant slog of work exhausts you and you'll need some time to rest and recharge by avoiding everything that makes you feel pressured at work. It is time to take to take a break from work if you've been working on a huge project for a long time.

If you want to get away from the workplace for a few minutes, you can leave the office to breathe in fresh air and enjoy an espresso. In this way, you'll feel more relaxed and full of energy when you return to work.

Talk to people

Participate in small gatherings, especially during lunchtime and make an effort to meet your colleagues as best you can. Enjoy an iced tea or coffee with a few of them who you believe are similar to the ways you think. A bit of interaction can be beneficial in establishing a good working relationship with them.

You may choose to talk to just one or two people if you're in larger groups, and then talk to them , if you are unable to converse with a lot of individuals at once. This method will allow you to avoid getting the stigma of being reserved in the workplace to a large degree.

Take Time Alone Time Alone

There are numerous spaces in all offices at one time or another, to talk about personal matters or work that requires complete concentration. Ask for help from one of your colleagues in finding the right spot.

Keep in mind that you should have the quiet area when doing something that is very crucial. You will only be able to give your best effort when you put all of your energy and effort in the task at hand.

Chapter 4: Overall Survival in Office of Extroverts

Being an introvert, you must learn how to live in the workplace that is not your ideal environment, however, you have to accept it due to specific situations. If a particular workplace is designed for people who are extroverts, it is definitely difficult for introverts to progress in the workplace.

Introverts must be aware of the best ways to manage a workplace filled with extroverts, especially in an open layout office. In this section, you'll be taught basic strategies and tricks to use as an introvert to make life easier for you and be successful in this type of environment.

Use Comfortable Workspace

People who are introverts do better in a place where they feel relaxed because there are a lot of things they observe around them, and their presence can make them feel happy.

If, for instance, you love flowers, then you can have some blooms in a vase in your living space. If you are a book lover it's an excellent idea to store your most-loved books placed in your work space.

By doing these things, you feel at home and the more at ease you feel in your work environment, the higher your chance of success be.

Enjoy a few hours of solitude

There are a lot of distinct variations we can see between extroverts versus introverts. the most prominent one is the fact that interaction with other people. This can boost the energy of extroverts, while being alone gives introverts a sense of energization.

Being in a crowd in the workplace can drain you of a lots of energy, and it is essential to recharge your batteries. The best method to do this is to find a peaceful area where there isn't people around and where you can sit and sit for anywhere between fifteen and twenty minutes.

Plan to eat lunch by yourself during break, as it is the perfect time to relax in solitude. You may also decide to stay in your cabin when there's nobody around, and recover all your vitality in the solitude, as this is a very important thing to take care of prior to returning to work.

Create a Friend with a Similar Minded

It's simple for introverts to have the conversation going with just an individual at. Make an effort to establish a connection with any of your colleagues who are similar to you at work. It's best if it becomes friendship since having a buddy can make you feel more at ease in meetings , or any other gatherings.

Be sure to cherish your connection with that person since you're not likely to meet someone that thinks in the same way as your own in the world where extroverts rule all over the world.

Accept the role of Leader

A lot of great people throughout past have been deemed introverts. The list includes Isaac Newton to Albert Einstein as well as Bill Gates to Mark Zuckerberg. The achievements of the above individuals shows us that introversion shouldn't be a barrier for us in the event that we wish to accomplish the highest level of success in our lives.

Introverted leaders are always proven to produce better results than extroverts due to their ability to listen as a strength . They are also skilled at analyzing the ideas of their team and implementing them more efficiently.

Harvard Business School research has also shown that introverted leaders are able to better discern what's happening inside the heads and hearts of team members, and how productive this can be.

Do not hesitate to take on the challenge when you are asked to assume an important role in your leadership. Being an introvert, you are able to make use of your strengths and demonstrate your leadership skills by focusing upon what the team members can accomplish by understanding the needs of your team.

Be selective when attending meetings.

If you believe it's not important to go to the event, you're able to skip the event. It is possible to save your time and energy by investing it to be productive within your daily activities.

Only attend meetings that you cannot afford to miss for example, when the boss calls you to an urgent meeting or when the project/operations manager contacts everyone to give a crucial meeting.

Your main goal is to be increasing your performance within the group because being an introvert, you won't perform well in meetings with strong ideas or sharing of comments since that's not your forte but you can demonstrate that you're more efficient and effective as a committed team member and impress your bosses.

Do you prefer meeting style that is suited to You

Meetings can be a challenge generally speaking for introverts, particularly when a an extensive number of staff are involved. Many organizations have begun using the strategy of starting meetings without words, but an unwritten memo of a few pages which is given to everyone who attends. At these meetings, there is a complete silence unless the entire group has read the memo and is aware of the primary purpose that the conference.

This is great for introverts as it helps keep everyone's attention on what the gathering is about and what's to be discussed instead of focusing on irrelevant issues. This way , a large amount of energy is conserved and utilized for productive tasks.

Another great idea for holding meetings for introverts is to hold them in smaller groups rather than a bigger group, because when you are in the presence of a lesser numbers of participants, an introvert will feel happier sharing your thoughts and let everyone know your ideas.

Stay connected with Co-Workers

You'd like to sit whole day sitting at your desk , trying to focus on your job as an introvert. You do not want to know the activities of your coworkers. doing.

While it's beneficial, but maintaining a relationship to your coworkers is essential because you're working for an organization and may require help from anyone in a situation you aren't able to manage due to a inexperience or lack of knowledge.

Some people think it's a unnecessary to check in with their colleagues however they overlook the fact that keeping in touch with all the people in the office will be beneficial in the end. It's not necessary to go and entertain them , or develop an enduring relationship with all of them.

Take a just a few minutes and make a point of saying hello to every coworker and talk about if there's something you need to discuss about your work or ongoing project. It is a good idea to do this at least once the day, whenever you're at work, and it will result in positive results surfacing.

Use Noise Canceling Headphones

In the event of having to deal constantly with environmental stimulants and constant digital distractions for a prolonged periods, introverts discover themselves in a bind.

If your office is filled with the sounds of people's voices everywhere, making it difficult to concentrate which means you're unable to concentrate on your job. Naturally, this will negatively impact your productivity in the event that you fail to get rid of the distractions.

Utilize a pair of headphones that block noise to block all distracting sounds from coming into your ears, so you will be able to work in a focused manner.

Find a Peaceful Work Space

It's a fact that introverts are more imaginative when they work in a serene atmosphere, regardless of which area they work in because their brains are filled with energy and they make use of it to create amazing outcomes.

It is possible working in a tranquil area where there is no background noise and you can have the possibility to work in absolute silence during the day, but this isn't possible all times, particularly in offices with huge open floors.

If you are facing the issue of working in a noisy or noisy work environment and aren't able to focus on your task at all you should discuss your issue in front of your supervisor and be sure to explain the situation. When your manager is friendly and is aware of the situation, they will allow you to have an uncluttered area in which to do your work.

Fake the Extroversion

There are times where you're in a position in which the power of extroversion prevails and it is inevitable to behave as an extrovert. What you aren't able to perform as an introvert could be accomplished with a little effort, by displaying an extroverted attitude.

All you have to do is to figure out how to act like an extrovert, even though you're trying to appear like one and are facing opposition because you're going against your own nature, however it will be beneficial ultimately.

You must manage things carefully and allow yourself to recharge your batteries regularly because the more you behave in the mindset of an extrovert more mental energy you'll be losing.

Excel in Sales and Marketing

While sales and marketing is not the best job for introverts, one does need to be aware all strategies that will allow them to succeed as an introvert, by creating sales in any field exactly like an extrovert.

You'll learn some useful tips that can help you improve your effectiveness as a marketing or salesperson and reach your goals.

Manage different people according to their needs

The most common mistake introverts make in sales is that they don't examine people according to their own perceptions of which one is part of what nature , and which thing will be the most appealing to them.

It's clear that different people you meet don't respond to you the same way due to the fact that they differ from each other , and have different moods and settings in the moments you are with them. This means that you need to be aware of this and speak to everyone in a manner that is appropriate for them.

Get a handle on your Fear

Becoming fearless is vital to succeed, because it helps you become stronger and more able to take on tough situations and conquer any challenge. If you are afraid of talking about angry customers think about the things that can cause you to be nervous in this situation and discover how to stay in a calm state and keep things in check.

Try doing something every day that makes you feel anxious. Do it in the hope that you can accomplish it, but certain circumstances won't allow you to complete it. When you begin to reduce the fear you feel, you will gain confidence in yourself to face the challenges and turn them into feasible.

Enjoy time in public

Spend as much time out in the public areas as you can. In this means you'll have the opportunity to meet people with different opinions and the variety of people that you meet and improve your ability to be of how to deal with different individuals. You'll also increase confidence in yourself and ultimately help you in your work. it's not possible to perform well in sales if you are not confident.

Find Passion

Ease or difficulty of anything is all about our thoughts and how we see it. When we are driven about something, we naturally create the energy to pursue it and take on any challenge to achieve it. It is essential to be enthusiastic about the product or service that you've got to offer your customers.

It diverts your attention away from what the person listening to you might be thinking, and allows you to concentrate more on what offers are available to the customer. The more enthusiasm and passion you exhibit during your conversation, the simpler it is of keeping your listener interested in the conversation, and consequently greater the chance of selling would be.

Stay busy

If you're working continuously and your mind is constantly focused, and this can help you keep the negative thought from coming in your head, or any negative emotions you may experience as a result of having a difficult time in sales.

When results don't meet your expectations You must be engaged in a work to avoid getting frustrated. It is important to remain optimistic about your job and never lose faith in your.

Keep a positive attitude

Trust in your company and its product, and confidence in your company since without it you can't speak with confidence about anything and this is a crucial thing for sales.

Be confident in your abilities to succeed. Don't forget to follow up to your customers until they're either required to accept the offer or submit complaints about the offer.

Work with others

If you're unable to sell your business on a regular basis, and no strategy or trick is working, it's time to work with your team members. The result is if you go through back-to-back defeats as an introvert, you will become more introverted, and suffer from extreme anxiety.

Help other salespeople and attempt to make a sale for them. This way, you are more likely to succeed since you have nothing to lose, and you are able to are able to work hard with no pressure.

When you see positive results from working with another person it is possible to regain your foam, which can help you to steer things to the proper direction for yourself.

We Value Every Customer

Staying in contact with all customers who are who are in your lead, regardless of whether they're potential customers or not.

Sometimes, you don't know what the sales are going to come from, and it comes from a location you never expected it to be coming from. This method keeps your momentum going and you hopeful to see positive outcomes.

In public, you can speak

Improving your public speaking abilities is a huge benefit to you in sales because it will increase your confidence and eliminate the anxiety because you are an introvert.

There are many opportunities to interact through the opportunity to participate in any public speaking event to talk about the things that the audience is there for.

It is beneficial for you to increase confidence, especially when you need to convince people of something, and this will eventually allow you to persuade others.

Chapter 5: Career Networking Tips

While networking to find an employment opportunity or in developing the career can be difficult for all, introverts are likely to have greater difficulties because they must meet strangers and develop a productive relationship with their peers.

As an introvert , you must to be aware of how to interact with those you haven't met and having a memorable conversation with them.

Today, things aren't as complicated as they were in the past because of the technological advances. There is no need to go to huge seminars or have a meeting face to face with people. Thanks to social media as well as various other platforms, it is easy to communicate with individuals from different fields and collect the information that you need.

Due to your interactions in the digital age, you may need to attend to people or be invited to an interview to get a better chance This is the reason you'll need to have professional networking skills to make it through working life.

Here are some suggestions that you can employ to create healthy connections and boost the number of professionals who are relevant to your field on your list.

Be Realistic

Find what strengths are within you and create targets for yourself which you can easily reach.

It's simpler to accomplish smaller goals than more ambitious ones. As an introvert, you should be aware of the number of people you can meet at the same time, since meeting a huge numbers of people can cause difficulties for you.

Do not be afraid to seek help

Maintaining a positive attitude towards learning and being able to ask other people about things that you are unsure of is a practice that will lead you closer to meeting your goals. Do this and you will develop this habit that will not be hesitant when you require guidance on something that is important.

There are those who believe it's not worth the time to offer advice to others, however there's no shortage of experts in any profession who would love to assist others when they're facing trouble. It's all about selecting the right person to share what you're facing.

Join Online Group

In your professional life , you have to deal with many ups and downs and it's your professional colleagues who could offer you advice from their experiences that could help you.

It's a good idea to join an online group that is on Facebook and LinkedIn which gives you the chance to interact with fellow professionals in your field. Also, you can pick like-minded people to engage with.

It is essential to be involved regularly in these groups, and be aware of what other members are sharing to gain insight by their stories. It is also possible to discuss your experiences in the event that you've got one, and allow others to speak about it.

Ask Questions

Learning from others is possible if you are aware of the point they are trying to convey and the pertinent questions you can ask them.

Being able to listen better than an introvert can give you an advantage over the rest of us and you'll be able to reap the advantage of it during the networking gatherings.

Take note of everyone's thoughts and respond with enthusiasm and then ask questions if it is necessary. This will help ensure that your participation is prominent at the gathering and people is likely to remember your name for a many years to come.

Create Contact List

Make sure to keep contact information such as contact number, email address, accounts or LinkedIn address in case you meet people you haven't met before at a networking event , as following up is essential following a meeting with people who you have never met before.

Sending them a brief message, telling them your great experience with them, and that you would like to see them again in the near future. They are sure to give you an enthusiastic response, and your interactions will yield the results you're hoping for.

Utilize Social Profiles

Making a profile on a social network allows others to get to know you. This allows companies that want to work with you, or who are in a mutual advantage with you, are able to discover you.

On these profiles, you are able to showcase your abilities, your previous professional experiences, and anything else that is important to others may not be able to see in your resume.

Aim for Proactive Action

One of the traits of people who are successful is the fact that they organize their plans ahead of time to minimize the chance of failure to a minimal. Being an introvert it is vital to plan your tasks in advance and plan for the various forthcoming events you are required to go to.

Note important information for yourself on the paper along with any other questions you'd like to ask. This means you will not forget any important points you wish to talk about.

Talk about You

Do not make them feel like you're interrogating them by asking questions back and forth but do try to share some of your personal details every now and then. it will ensure that they do not forget what you said to them when the event is over.

Being an introvert, it's likely that you're not keen on letting people know about your life, especially it's difficult for you to share personal information with people, but you won't make strong connections in your business networking without sharing information about yourself and let others know that you.

Use Contacts to Meet New People

There are people that you don't have a connection to, but you would like to meet them, and the best way to reach them is through mutual contacts.

Ask your contacts if anyone has any knowledge of the particular person, There is a chance that someone knows or has had a conversation with that person. You can then be introduced easily.

It is actually a mutual contact rule that you can apply to your network, especially through social networks, and it has proven to be highly efficient on social media platforms.

It has been discovered in an interview that the majority of applicants get great jobs because of a recommendation. Maintaining contact with the entire group on a regular basis allows you to learn about something fast and you aren't able to miss an opportunity to be considered for a great job or an opportunity that's right to you.

Do it every day

There is no need to wait around for occasions to be planned for you to take advantage of networking opportunities , but you can take advantage of these opportunities on your own every day at work by engaging with your colleagues . In this means you can improve your skills each day.

Invite your colleagues to lunch or get together during office hours to discuss the things you're experiencing in your work and learn something new they've got to share with you.

Tips to be a successful and attractive person

It isn't easy to meet everyone, but it causes extra stress for introverts as they're already not great in meeting new people, and encountering someone from a different gender may be quite a challenge for them.

If you're looking to go out on a date , especially the first time as an introvert, the process could be quite difficult for you. You're thinking about what you should wear, how to be wearing and what your experience will be for you.

Many introverts are extremely anxious due to their anxiety about what they'll be saying in the course of conversation. It's not possible to ignore your introversion in the event that you decide to date one, but there are a few ways to make your first meeting successful.

Choose the place you are most familiar with

It is vital to know you pick the right place to meet at, if you visit a place that you're not familiar with and your focus is likely to be diverted to becoming accustomed to the new surroundings. In the end, you will not be able focus on the date in a proper manner and it is possible that the event will be ruined.

Pick a place you've been to several times in the past and are familiar with every corner and crevice. For instance, if you plan to meet in a coffee place that you normally frequent and know all the details there will not only assist you to remain in a safe position, but will also allow you to arrive at the right time.

Practice by rehearsing

Doing some practice before stepping into something that seems difficult to you, could be beneficial to get the desired results. The first time you meet someone is unlike anything you've ever had before, so practicing the questions you'll have to discuss or general questions that you will need to address can ease the anxiety you feel.

Take a partner along and practice with the person you are with. Discuss how you should respond to certain situations and take their comments about your facial expressions and body language. This will help you avoid making mistakes that could be harmful for your date . You will also know how to conduct an a memorable conversation when you first meet.

Meet for Short Time

Although first dates don't last very long since the two individuals know very little or nothing about each other , you must ensure that you get together for only a few minutes.

With that in mind, make sure that your partner is invited to join you for coffee or a drink. This will ensure that your date is going to last a shorter amount of time and you won't need to be concerned about it.

The way you plan your date isn't putting too much pressure on you . This is a problem you will have to meet when you decide to have dinner or lunch. If you are later satisfied that the event went well and you're enjoying the time, you could suggest that you extend the date.

Don't make too many changes

If you are thinking you must buy a new outfit for your date or brand new glasses or wristwatch You can pick the one you think looks the best in that particular moment , but there's no reason to make modifications that you're not comfortable with.

Don't wear clothes that do not fit your personality, since you might look uncomfortable and not create a positive impression.

There is no need to be at yourself in a way that makes you feel uncomfortable when you're with your romantic partner in a dress you've never have before or with something that you're not used to. Try to raise your confidence level by wearing the same clothes you wear every day.

Ask questions that are open-ended

Avoid asking closed end questions. Also, always inquire questions that require an explanation. This will allow your partner to talk more and you can listen. Inquiring open-ended questions help your friend realize that you're taking an interest in them and want to learn more about them.

Be cautious about one thing to ensure that you don't make your partner feel as if you're interrogating them. Do not keep asking questions repeatedly, instead, you should be able to tell some of your personal details after a couple of questions on what the discussion is about.

It is important to be prepared to respond to questions too, since should someone ask questions about something you're not prepared to answer and explain, it's not an encouraging signal from your side. Be sure to talk about your job and any other obligations you're currently engaged in, however, don't divulge any details about your private life which isn't required to discuss.

Pick an environment that is interesting

If you're worried about engaging in conversations with someone who's close to being a stranger It is best to pick an area where you are required to speak less since your partner's attention is captivated by the surrounding all the time. There should be something exciting to look at or do which helps you to avoid the small talk, and ensures you have a great time.

If you're a fan of soccer, it is possible to get together at a soccer game or meet on the golf course if you are a fan of the sport. Going swimming with your partner at an interesting location is an excellent alternative.

In addition to playing games, fascinating spots to consider include amusement parks, zoos or a museum. It is important to make your decision wisely as dating is about learning new what each person are able to enjoy.

Be Honest

Many people are unsure how to talk about their introversion before going to meet someone first-time and wish to develop an excellent relationship with the person. If that's the case, then be sure to inform them that you are an introvert with a feature and then explain how you have used this trait in a positive way in your own life and used it to your advantage, not as weak point.

If your relationship is ongoing it is possible to cover it up for a few dates, but if you are required to attend an event or social event with your partner it could be revealed. It would be difficult for you to admit that you are feel guilty, so it is best to be honest and open about your character in confidence.

Stay Optimistic

You may be looking for a suitable partner to go out with or even in your personal life, there are times when things don't go to be the way you expected but there's no need to be frustrated as there's always a way when there is a desire.

It's possible that your date has an unlikable person who you didn't know in your conversations with them via phones, social media or other channels. If you decide, following the first meeting, that this isn't the person you're looking for, be truthful and inform them that you're an individual with distinct ideas and preferences that they do and you have no common ground with them.

The goal of dating is finding out about the interests or beliefs that both partners have in common. when there are no or only a few items discovered, there is no reason to spend time and effort in trying to maintain an affair that could end sooner or later in a disastrous and heartbreaking manner.

Keep your eyes open and continue looking for the person you're looking for to be with, utilizing the guidelines and tips that you were taught as an introvert to dating. You will eventually meet someone who has a personality that is compatible to yours, and you will make a great pair that everyone is awed by.

Don't be frustrated

Both bad and good experiences are normal part of life. Everyone experiences each of them in different phases of their lives. You need to be tough enough to face every circumstance that you encounter.

Being an introvert, you possess an impressive memory, which is good for you. However, in certain situations, if there are just bad memories that have been associated with you from the time you were together, it's difficult to erase the details and it can be an unpleasant experience.

Instead of not letting the negatives from the relationship experience you just experienced, occupy your mind constantly, focus on the things that appear to be positive in the. Be aware of the mistakes you made and the crucial lessons you took away from them will aid you in your journey and avoid making the same mistakes on the next time you meet.

What is the best way to Make Friends

Introverts are eager to make friends for a life full of happiness and enjoyment similar to extroverts however, things can be difficult for them since meeting new people can make them uncomfortable . They have no idea where to initiate conversations.

However, this doesn't mean as an introvert , you shouldn't make friends and live life just like everyone else. All you have to do is accept the difficulties that you will face in the course of making new friends.

Being an introvert doesn't cause you to be a nuisance or convince them that you're not a great friend. There are numerous qualities that you possess that are superior to others because of your introverted nature and people would like to see the same qualities in every friend they meet. Introverts, for instance, have a strong sense of loyalty, provide the right advice, they are dedicated, innovative, and so on.

This chapter you'll not only discover the strategies and strategies to follow in making new friends, but also the skills to create stronger bonds with your friends.

Very Little Interaction

When people gather for a social gathering, they typically place people in two categories depending on the type of interactions they've had one group is friendly while the other one is rude.

It doesn't mean you should be giving all the time you can and engage in an enjoyable conversations with them to present your self as a person who is friendly and at large gatherings, it may be impossible. The best thing could you do instead is introduce yourself to them and that's enough to demonstrate that you are an open-minded person.

This small exchange could be beneficial in establishing an enduring relationship with the person who you will meet again and then transforming into a solid friendship.

Speak to strangers

Being an introvert, you are likely to be a weak participant when it comes to social interactions. If you are in this circumstance, it is important to learn to be more social with people. Similar to how you worked to enhance every skill you have learned throughout your life, it is possible to enhance your social abilities.

It is not necessary to travel to locations where you'll meet new friends to socialize with, however, you should be prepared to speak to strangers who appear in your everyday life. It's not required to establish a connection with them, but this habit will increase your confidence.

The most important thing is improving your ability to converse with strangers in various social settings. Another way to take your abilities further is to emulate people whose style of social interaction is amazing to you.

Be aware of others and discover who is the best at the art of socializing and observe how they attract all with their unique style of speaking.

Don't Talk About Controversial

Consider the things that appeal to you most, or what are your personal preferences and likes because you must discover people with something in common with your views, beliefs or other things you enjoy. It is essential to identify common interests since they create the basis for an enduring friendship.

If you're in contact with people you have never met before. Be sure to stay clear of talking about issues which are controversial or linked to some issue. It is possible to have your say on political and religious topics or express an enthusiasm for them however, if you engage in deeper conversations without understanding the viewpoint of the person or group can stoke the discussion.

It is only possible only if you're with someone or an organization of people who share a the same ideology, which you are aware of.

Find common interests

It is a known fact that it is much easier to establish friendships with people who share a similar interest with you, as this can create a bond between two individuals and they want to learn more about one another and spend more time with each other.

If you go to the seminar or computer class, lecture or join the book club, you stand a good chance of finding like-minded individuals who have many of the same interests as you.

The best part is that you will have plenty to discuss when you talk with other people in these places and you don't need to be concerned about making small conversation with people.

You're already aware of the purpose of these chats and can begin the conversation by asking a few more formal questions.

Participate in Social Events

It is important to build strong friends who can assist you through difficult times, because friends in need are actually a friend however, such individuals are rare and could be great friends. You don't have to fret, just go to social gatherings and get togethers where you'll be able to meet new people.

You shouldn't miss any occasion, especially if you realize that you've got a small number or no people in your life. You must expand your social circle to open the door of prosperity for yourself.

Because of an introverted nature You won't be able to find it easy to join social gatherings that are filled with strangers. The best thing could you do? to a group of people who can introduce you to strangers. This way you can be socialized as you make new acquaintances will feel easy for you.

Use Proper Body Language

It's not only that you need to greet all people at a social gathering, but you could also make others to notice you when you make use of a warm body language.

If you are walking or standing with your head down with your hands in your pockets and your hands in your pocket, nobody will want to meet you due to the fact that you've adopted an unattractive posture. If you're willing to let people approach them and talk to them, all you have to do is alter your body language.

Keep your head up and straight back with shoulders in a parallel line and put a look on your face. This kind of body language will make you appear confident, and it is sure to inspire people to hang with you at any social gathering that you attend.

A common mistake introverts make that inhibits body language friendly and puts them into the defensive position is crossing their arms and legs. It shows that you do not want to speak to anyone, but just watch or listen to what's happening around you.

Engage in Conversations

For the majority of introverts, the biggest concern is how to initiate conversations when they meet someone new and often aren't able to come up with an ideas. This is a problem when it comes to getting to know new people and becoming great acquaintances.

Start the conversation by sharing something about yourself, as this will signal to the other person that you're looking forward to talking with them, and as a consequently, they will respond appropriately.

It's not necessary to talk about something extremely personal or talk about a bad moment you've experienced Let them know that you're to this gathering to the very first time and tell them how you feel about being part of this group.

Engage in Conversations with Others

People love to talk about themselves or discuss their thoughts with other people. If you ask them a closed-ended question isn't a good choice because it's not likely to result in an appropriate conversation.

Always ask an open-ended question to allow them to talk about the question you asked. It it also lets them know that you're interested in learning more about the person you asked.

If you're meeting people who is for the first time get their opinion on the things that everyone gathered to discuss.

If you're meeting with someone for the third time, it is advisable to ask them "How do you feel?", but if you've had several meetings previously inquire about their plans for the weekend and the places they like to go to.

Keep in touch

If you are trying to make acquaintance with someone, it's important to keep in contact regardless of whether you contact them or send them messages on social media. You have to inform them in one method or another that you would like to meet them in the future.

Invite them to join you for the restaurant or lunch at your house or at your home, or you could also plan an event somewhere different from the spot you met the last time.

Even though this is just a beginning, there is a lot that is required to transform this relationship into an actual friendship, it is crucial and each that you expect to come in the near future will depend on how you manage the initial phase.

You should mention a idea in lieu of asking to meet up with you. For instance, you could mention that you plan to watch a film this weekend and would like them to join you.

Be Prepared Before You Move

It's not the case that all the moment you'll be making efforts to connect with people but it's also possible that someone will approach you in search of friendship through making a phone call or sending a message.

In this scenario, you could need to consider what you should do prior to deciding whether or not to respond, especially if you have not considered being friends with the person.

Be aware that you cannot make a decision on someone in a moment however, you should take time to get to know them to make a final decision. Therefore, you should try to engage in an interaction with them and get to get to know them better and inform them about yourself because this can give you an idea the possibility of creating any kind of chemistry.

Communicate intelligently

If you are an introvert, you may not be at ease all the time when talking on the phone. Messenger chat or text message is a different method of communication that you could make use of to keep in touch with the people you're building friendships with.

One thing to make sure of is whether the person you are talking to is interested in your conversations as you move deeper in building a rapport with them. Otherwise, you could waste your time since they may not take this seriously . At some point, they'll likely start to ignore you.

It is not something that can be achieved overnight, but it develops like a tiny plant growing from the seed. It requires proper nourishment through sunlight that is filled with love as well as water interest.

Be prepared for the difficult times that you will encounter at first and remember that things will improve getting easier as you progress in your relationship.

Learn how to combat frustration and continue searching for the things you require. There are instances when the results do not go like you expected, but don't give up hope and remain positive since there's always someone who is waiting who can be an excellent friend.

Chapter 6: Party Survival Tactics

There's a widespread belief that introverts aren't a good choice being in a crowd and do not enjoy parties. However, it's not true in reality.

People who are introverted have a lower level of time when compared to people who are able to use the power of extroversion. However, that does not mean they cannot enjoy a night out or get together like an person who is extroverted. It's merely a issue of maintaining an appropriate level of energy. The more energy they can store within their bodies, the more able they is.

If you are an introvert, then you must understand the importance of your interaction in any social setting and how to survive in it without losing energy completely and becoming exhausted.

In this chapter, you'll learn easy methods to help you navigate any event without pain feasible and to enjoy every aspects of the party as any extrovert would.

Have a companion

It's a good idea to travel with someone who will help you spend a few minutes of time in peace by distracting the other and locating a place to spend quiet time. Your close friends could be able to help you and help you get out of trouble when you're caught in.

There is a huge advantage when you're joined by an extrovert companion at the event as it is frequently observed that when two individuals who are introverted and another with an extrovert personality traits are paired together and they are able to meet the needs of each other when needed and the extrovert could make it possible to the introverts for a way out from social gatherings.

However, an introvert might suggest innovative solutions to resolve a problem their extrovert colleagues since they can be observant.

Find a spot to be Solitude

The first thing you need to take care of is to find a space to yourself, where you can take a break and recharge your batteries in case you are exhausted at any point in the evening. It is easy to do this even if you're having a the party in your home, but it's an enormous concern if you're in the home of someone else.

Prepare yourself mentally in case you're invited to an event in a venue that you're not familiar with. It is necessary to put in an extra effort and ask assistance from someone else to locate an area that is quiet and where you can get back to your energetic level. The most suitable spots are the corridors, balconies bathrooms, kitchens, or any other room that is empty.

Be aware of all options in your mind, because in the event that one option is not accessible, you may choose the alternative. Make sure that you do not enter an area where entry for everyone is restricted and only do this if you are completely aware of the area.

Be aware of your energy Level

If you are planning to have fun until the very end, you must be cautious concerning your level of energy, and try to keep them going with short breaks. Every time you feel that you're in need of recovery then you must take action immediately.

If you notice that you're getting tired Try to stop conversations with people or the group that you're in. You can then make the excuse of something that you must do for instance, making a phone call to someone or searching for a friend in the group.

If you aren't paying the attention of this and remain stuck in the conversation for a longer, you'll are in trouble because you'll lose all the energy and be forced to choose other than to leave the event promptly.

Help with Parties Arrangements

If you're looking to stay away from the group chatter as you're not in the mood to spend your time or speak to everyone at the gathering You can play the lead in helping to get rid of everything by heading to the location where physical assistance is required.

Offer a helping hand in the kitchen while you cook something, or assist with making choices or giving gifts to guests.

There's a shortage of individuals from all walks of life, who could be a part of the planning process. Make sure you are prepared for anything it is possible to do to help keep things running smoothly at the party. So, you'll be able to avoid from being in situations in which too much talk is required.

Know Who the Guests Are

Friends are great to spend time with. As many people you meet at the event you're attending more comfortable your life will be for an introvert. Imagine how challenging it is for you if you're at a gathering with a crowd with fewer or no people.

Find out who's coming to the party and who's not. It's an excellent idea to create a list of individuals who will be at the event. You'll be able to determine among those who are there you will know how many close people from your circle are attending and who are secure. This will assist you in making the choice of whether to attend the party or not.

Concentrate on Listening

Being an introvert, you have better listening than most people, and should utilize these skills more often than you converse with others. When you're engaged in conversation with people who are extroverts demonstrate through body expression that you are paying attention to them and are interested in what they have to say.

Try to talk as little as you can and conserve energy for yourself. Make sure you are aware of the subject and be sure to ask questions occasionally. In this way, you'll allow them to have more time to speak and will also let them feel like you're engaged in the discussion.

Make Your Choices

The types of parties that introverts tend to be comfortable with are those hosted at home, but it is important to be aware of the ways to survive to ensure that they can be utilized when needed.

The amount of time you've set for each person that you must interact with at the gathering is vital because you need to make plans according to. You'll know the amount of time you will devote to a specific group of people quickly and effectively.

If you are too involved with one individual or group of people during the event, you won't be able to connect with your fellow guests because you're an introvert, and your capacity for interaction isn't like the other. Also, you must take note of whom you are with at the event and whose relationship is more important to you.

Prioritizing your priorities is beneficial so that you don't miss contact with someone who has developed a solid connection with you, which could help you over the long term.

Plan when to leave

You are able to have a wonderful time and be able to enjoy every minute as long as you know about the exact time to go out and return to bed. Create a schedule and adhere to it to the letter.

Spend your time in quiet areas, according to your preference however, try not to stay there if you're at another's house. This can definitely disrupt your routine. If you're not adept in managing your time, you should follow the timetable of those who are adept at managing and socializing.

Chapter 7: Tips for Travel

An introvert's method of thinking and interpreting things is a bit different from other people's and this is the reason why many people do not understand those with this type of personality.

They believe that introverts would prefer to be in solitude and have no desire to travel or explore the world. This is a huge misconception because introverts are extremely attracted to long drives and are eager to explore new and exciting destinations.

Traveling can provide you with the most enjoyable experience as an introvert . you'll be able to recharge your mind when you take an break from the routine and spend time in the place you've had always wanted to go to for an extended period of time.

Learn here useful tips that will make your travel experience unforgettable and enjoyable for the rest of your life. Let's take a take a look at the things you need to remember prior to embarking for the adventure of a lifetime.

Keep a Travel Journal

It is a good idea to have a travel journal and note down your thoughts, especially when you're in a cafe or restaurant. coffee shop. This allows you to convey your feelings about the moment, regardless of whether you're feeling happy, excited or even scared.

It's finally time to feel and relax after a very busy day at work. You don't want to miss a second of it as it's the best time of your life.

Once you've written down your feelings and all the emotions you felt in your journal, it's ideal to revisit them at some point after you return from your trip.

Keep items that will help you Stay clear of Small Talk

It's difficult to engage in conversation with someone who is an introvert when you're traveling and you find ways to stay clear of this.

The simplest way to do this is by keeping the book you want to read, or use headphones to play music. The advantage of that is that you won't be rude in this manner and you won't need to worry about the awkwardness of small conversation.

Don't be afraid to travel alone

The introverts don't have to travel in a group or one of their peers to enjoy their time , but they do know how to have fun and keep them entertained even when they're on their own. The advantage of traveling by yourself is that you have the freedom to independently do whatever you want to that you like without interfering.

If you believe there's something lacking that you can enjoy with a group or a partner, you may be able to meet with a few locals and you might be able to meet someone who will spend time with you and imparts knowledge which can benefit you.

Make Sure to Take Your Camera with You

The majority of introverts enjoy photography or videography. Bring your digital camera and camera with you to make the most to capture a breathtaking scene so that it can become an irresistible memory of your excursion for the rest of your life.

Another advantage of being engaged in what you love in doing is the people who are around will not bother your enjoyment and you will be able to take your time and enjoy the moment.

Pick a hotel that is Conventional

You must be aware that any hotel could not be the best choice for you when you pick a smaller hotel where there is a lot of congestion in the places you circulate, you could quickly meet other travellers who are staying at the exact same place.

After a hectic and tiring journey, you're not in the mood to get to know people or let them know about your experiences. Therefore, it's better to be far from the busyness and enjoy your time alone, which allows you to regain the energy that you've lost. In this regard, consider looking for the largest hotel in which you feel completely alone and enjoy some peace at the end the day.

Relax and unwind.

If you have the chance to retreat, then it's perfect for you to be an introvert. Find a retreat group to do writing, yoga, meditation and painting or anything else you love the most.

It is a opportunity to get away from the usual distractions and let your mind, body and spirit to grow stronger. There is no need to be concerned about being lonely while you're on retreat since all of the participants have the same reason.

Eat in the room at times

If you're traveling in a foreign country, you'll be eating at restaurants from breakfast to dinner. And eating three meals during the day away from home could make you tired since you'll be having interactions with other people.

No matter if you're taking the trip with your buddies or by yourself, it's best to have room service in order to stay clear of socializing. Another good idea is to carry some food with you such as snacks so that you won't be feeling hungry all the time.

Watch for a while

The introverts lack energy when they travel frequently to different locations and at times, they're stressed. This is something you'd never want to occur for you. So be well-prepared and schedule some time to recharge yourself.

Enjoy a few minutes in an area cafe and relax watching the world go by and the people who walk through the area. The time spent in a quiet place makes you feel more relaxed and energetic which allows you to explore more of the area and makes your trip more enjoyable.

Explore while walking

The majority of introverts aren't keen to take a walk on the streets of a city especially when the area is completely unfamiliar to them.

Walking tours give an experience unlike anything else can't be had by using transportation, as you have the chance to know more about the city and its inhabitants.

If you come across something you're not familiar with Don't be afraid to ask someone else about it since as a tourist, you should not miss the chance to find out something interesting or interesting you find.

Be careful when speaking to new People

Being an introvert doesn't mean you're anti-social It's just that you'd like to have a moment to you.

While it's good to engage in conversation with strangers and learn about them, engaging in lengthy conversations with them could lead to an invitation or offer you may not like. Thus, it is essential to be sure to ensure that your conversation doesn't drag on and drains your time or energy.

People who are introverts have a hard time to say no, but you are expected to be able to be able to say "no" right away to something that you do not feel at ease with. In the end, you're in a an unfamiliar environment with strangers, and anything can occur that you were not anticipating.

Make sure you choose your destination carefully

Experimenting with new and unique locations is great, but you must be sure to choose your destination carefully based on your level of energy.

Don't make the mistake of going to a distant location away from the hotel you're staying at, which means much time and energy may be wasted.

Make a plan for will determine what day, and which locations you must visit and determine how long it will take. In this means you are conscious of all things and can manage your time according to.

Choose New Locations

While it is great to travel to cities in which there are family members or friends because you will be able to enjoy and have a great time however, as an introvert you travel to be alone solely, you must pick a destination that you aren't surrounded by people.

One hand, you'll be unable to spend your experiences with in the new location, but at the same time, you'll be observing a brand new world with plenty to discover and find fascinating items to share with everyone after returning after your journey.

CHAPTER 8: Going from Introvert to Extrovert in Six Simple Steps

An introvert won't transform into an extrovert in a single day. However there are a variety of steps they can use to bring out their extrovert side.

1. Be open-minded

It's difficult to discern from yourself a character characteristic that you view as negative. Every time introverts see generalization extroverts complex, loud and insane.' Explore the possibility of extroverts as something positive. Take a look at the many people you have met who are extroverts and with whom you remain friends with, or even with pay attention and respect. You can identify the traits that you admire in these individuals. You'll realize that a significant portion of them have related to their extrovert personality. Therefore, being an extrovert doesn't mean at the worst thing to be.

2. Receive Opposite Behaviors

Try to be an extrovert until you reach the moment when it is all the more widely to you. When you work, take the chance to draw attention to you and your work area by placing pictures on the divider or in a collection of rolls in your workspace. Food items that are visible can draw more attention than you expected, especially because we're talking about free food here!

3. Act the Part

The majority of actors on stage and screen are extremely shy. They are the only ones who accept the role of an anecdote or mimic a real person and discover that the possibility of a different persona lets them become more outgoing. For instance, it is apparent that he can appear to be quite modest at certain occasions, yet he's one of Britain's top entertainers. Even if you're not typically cordial You possess the skills to entertain and show off your skills to impress people. Think back to your school drama or drama classes and the way you used them to immerse yourself in the work. Do not think that you're not real, you've erred in putting the phrase 'demonstrate it until the point that you believe it' into the training.

4. Gain From Others

In any unintentional grouping of individuals, there'll be a mix of extroverts and introverts. There are extroverts across your personal and professional networks, no matter if you're part of your social group of old university friends or your work group. Be attentive to these individuals to observe what they do in and how they interact with you, and benefit from their activities.

5. Know Yourself

Examine your identity to determine discover what makes you different from different from other people. You could be a similar sexuality, within the same age group and of the same social class with someone and but be completely different from the other. Don't expect that, since you're in the an identical group of statistics as males, you act exactly like them. Be aware of what is interesting about you. can help you understand the way you interact with people like managers, colleagues, questioners and spotters. This will help you identify and separate areas of your personality that could enhance.

6. Support other introverts

Think about your options for the possible introvert being referred to isn't you, but rather it's a coworker. Anyone who has been a successful group leader particularly one who seats numerous gatherings will tell you to watch closely at introverts and try to incorporate them into your group, because they're unlikely to be able to discuss. Provide security to the quieter members of the group in a way of reminding more extrovert people of their inclusiveness. Let introverts talk. When someone is about to impede or talk to someone else, ask that they remain calm and listen and ask that the person in question remain in conversation. It's your you and, in this way, to your greatest advantage, allow everyone to speak."

You are an introvert? This is How to Tell

A person who is introverted is often thought of as a calm contemplative, reserved person. They do not seek out extra attention or social interactions because these occasions can make introverts feel depleted and exhausted.

We know that these traits of personality don't come from big or in the bank. Introverts may have elements of extroversion that are part of their personality. They might enjoy following the stages or throwing parties. Extroverts might prefer a bit more privacy at times and prefer working alone when they really have to concentrate.

Personality traits of introverts

Here are some of the most common traits of introversion that are common to people:

Then you'll be able to slow down and get your

Being at home on your own is a pleasure and not exhausting. The moments of quiet are essential to the wellbeing of an introvert and joy. No matter if you're relaxing or engaging in a sport, being alone can be a great source of relaxation. People who are introverts often like reading, cultivating writing, creating and gaming, watching films or performing any other activity that is performed in solitude.

Social interactions deplete you

While extroverts don't want to be able to resist an evening out on Friday with friends, introverts are aware they've exhausted themselves and need to recharge their batteries. It doesn't mean that all introverts end into a lonesome crowd -they are able to and do appreciate them just as an extrovert however, at the end of a long day introverts require a break to recharge and rejuvenate.

You are a fan of working in a team

If a group activity is intimidating or unpleasant, then you could be an introvert. People who are introverts usually do most effectively when they work in solitude. This allows introverts to be focused and produce top-quality work. It's not to say that introverts can't be effective with other people; they just prefer to be alone and focus on what they need to be done, rather than looking at the social aspect when working within a group.

The term "introvert" is commonly used to describe as a quiet, calm and thoughtful person. They do not seek out extra attention or social events since these activities can make introverts feel depleted and exhausted.

Extraverts and introverts may be differentiated based on how they replenish energy. The term "extrovert" is utilized more often as opposed to "extrovert." Introverts tend to gravitate towards small-scale environments that stimulate them They require the time to be alone in order to get their energy back. Extroverts recharge by socializing in a group.

We know that these characteristics didn't win big or even a bust. Introverts have aspects of extroversion in the form of their identity. They may enjoy following the stages or throwing parties. Extroverts might appreciate a little more privacy from time to time and would prefer to work on their own in times when they have to concentrate.

You've got a close circle of friends , and you like this as such

Do not make an introvert's small circle of acquaintances as a sign that they don't have friends or don't want to socialize. They like talking to individuals and becoming more acquainted with other people. They also prefer the intimacy of a small group of friends. A strong network of connections is the essential ingredient to happiness for introverts as demonstrated by one study.

You are curious and introspective.

It is possible to end up thinking or planning things out in your head long before you create the order of your activities or even lift a finger to change any thing. Introverts are very active in their inner perspective. They also tend to reflection and investigation. They are driven to look for their passions and are informed and well-read.

You are to blame for daydreaming for a tonne

People who are introverts frequently "escape" from their surroundings by meditating or giving their minds the time to drift away from what they need to be done. If you're one of them, this could be a method of leaving an environment that is disorganized or uncomfortable or stressful. It's a survival tool in a sense. However to other people it could seem as if you're not focused.

You favor composing over talking

You're more comfortable writing down your thoughts rather than talking about them in a way that's not your best, particularly when you're unprepared. You are keen to think about your response because your manner of correspondence is shrewd and professional. It is possible to continue conversations, but should decisions are vital you might need more time to think about and weigh your options to ensure you are confident that you are making the right choice.

You "feel" more

One study shows that introverts are likely to be deemed to have wretchedness. This could be due, as another research suggests, that introverts aren't as happy often as extroverts. It's unclear why introverts do not feel more content however it could be a lot to do with the way introverts perceive the joy. Introverts tend to have a more optimistic and an enthusiastic and positive direction. It isn't easy to attain this level of satisfaction continuously.

Introversion can be described as a range

Many people are not just extrovert or introverted. They're somewhere in between, possessing characteristics that are both. Certain traits could be more grounded that's why people can self-identify as introvert or an extrovert.

Your traits can play an important role in determining which side of the spectrum of personality. Studies have shown that those who are extroverted have a different reaction to dopamine, which is a chemical that is found in the reward system of your brain. Extroverts feel a rush of happiness or energy due to social interactions as a result of the mixture. People who are introverts experience a sense of overstimulation.

Your past can have a profound impact on your character and personality. It is possible to alter or slide a little within the duration of. It is possible to figure out ways to talk to others in a way that is different and benefit from the experience as an adult.

There is no reason to alter or modify your character. Whatever you do, your personality is an essential part of who you are.

The Introvert-Extrovert Connection: 3 Tips to make it work

Relationships between introverts and extroverts are very possible. Don't opposites pull in? Although it's enjoyable to control someone special to you might be but there are instances that two people just do not agree.

Do you have a way to control conflict in this kind of situation? What are the best ways to handle the introvert-extrovert connection? Find out about a few suggestions that are accommodating.

Tip 1: Recognize Each Others' Strengths.

While the introverts and extroverts might be, there should be respect between the two groups. The two groups should find out ways to be respectful of the other's perspective.

The introverts may be quiet but they also tend to generally be more attentive. Because they are less likely to draw attention to themselves they might be able to spot things that others do not.

Extroverts, on the other hand, are the mainstays of the gathering. They're determined and leave unforgettable impressions.

"Modify" your attitude towards anyone you see as contrary to yours. You'll be amazed at how you'll be able to see how much better your relationship will be when you have established an environment of respect for all.

Tip 2: Learn to Understand Each One's weaknesses.

A bit of persistence can go a long way. Create an introvert-extrovert partnership that works both parties should be aware of where one is defenceless. Not because that is where they are able to strike however, it is their cue to step in and help.

The importance of support is paramount to any partnership. Introverts are more likely to mix in at an event, and so extroverts must help push them to come out and make them feel comfortable with others.

Extroverts might not have the energy to reflection. Maybe introverts are able to achieve a bit of harmony.

Tips 3: Agree or Not Agree.

In general introverts and extroverts both have topics that they generally don't accept. In this case there isn't a preferred solution that can be reached to agree on an agreement.

The debate over who has a superior mind or is right won't help anyone. The result is more conflict. In settling for an agreement that everyone has had an act of respect.

As resentful as it may be sometimes, it's better than arguing with one another in the event of an issue of assessment or beliefs.

An introvert-extrovert bond can be extremely energizing. Much like any other relationships It is not without its high points as well as lows. The methods mentioned above might be the solution you're searching for, but they willat a minimum help to disperse a bit of the disagreement.

What are the main differences between Introverts and Extroverts?

What is the best way to recharge?

The most basic distinction between extroverts and introverts is the way they recharge. Extroverts recharge through being with other people. An introvert recharges through investing time alone or with one of their confided-in friends or two.

Who do you do you trust?

Extroverts will probably take to the phone when they are separated from their peers. They require someone to talk with about what's happening or not. They may be thought to be shy but they are bound to confide to a few people. They will likely consider their options before deciding to act or even discussing their thoughts with somebody.

Act or think, which is the one that gets things going?

The introvert has a tendency to be the first person to think. Introverts tend to observe situations prior to taking part. They will likely think of different possible outcomes before they take a decision or discuss the issues. Extroverts are individuals who are active. They usually need to think in terms of. They will likely to be unconstrained and move swiftly.

It's safe to say that you're chatty?

Extroverts view introverts as sexy and often overly talkative. Extroverts typically view introverts as rude or indifferent to social. The opposite is true. Extroverts must talk and interact with other people. Introverts tend to think before speaking. Some introverts are overwhelmed in group settings or gatherings. A reason why introverts are regarded as calm is that they remain quiet for a period of time during a conversation prior to speaking while extroverts are more likely to start speaking when they have a break.

What do you do when you are you are focused?

A person who is extroverts will likely to gather friends for activities or to increase their capacity. They could go shopping or locate a place where there are people. People who are introverts will always take a step back. They might go home and relax with a book or even watch a movie at home. Introverts may make one or two friends, but is likely to stay clear of groups until the pressure is less.

Everyone is either extrovert or introvert. But we all have a mix of both types of personality within us. Although there are plenty positives to being an introvert it is sometimes necessary to recognize your extrovert side. A greater degree of an extrovert can aid you in being at a higher level of engagement with your customers and potential clients.

Here are a few suggestions on how to accomplish it with less effort faster and more efficiently:

1. Adore your turf

Many introverts feel most at ease within their own environment. You can make it work, organize events at your home ground as often as you can, whether it's a last meal at the most loved restaurant and a delicious meal in your home for your date or even making a dash to your preferred place to relax for the time of a party.

This can help you make connections with other people in the same atmosphere. This will also assist you in becoming more comfortable speaking to others and leaving your comfortable zone.

2. Smile often and practice it.

The non-verbal cues you receive are more groundbreaking than you would think. It is preferential for other people to engage in conversations and approach them or to encourage them by smiling and looking. You can practice it in the city, in the grocery store, or almost everywhere other than there.

People associate happiness and pleasure by smiling. This can make prospective customers relax and become more relaxed around you, which makes an offer much more likely.

3. Practice, practice and practice

You can be a force for brief conversation with anyone including your barista or broker at any circumstance at any time throughout the day. If you are willing to try things that are unusual and the more comfortable you'll feel. In addition, you might be able to get some limits not too that far away!

On a regular basis, you should be engaging in conversation with people out of your familiar zone. "How are you doing this moment?" and then a quick follow-up with "What's your impression of (embed recent news or a particular theme)?" Start a conversation. The more you get comfortable to this, the more certain that you'll be able to perform it in systems management situations where it's actually necessary.

4. Permit re-charge time

A lot of introverts agree that although they enjoy (a small number of) individuals, they also require some time to recharge. If you're planning to do something that requires you to be extrovert, you should consider the time you spend in your own home.

5. Join Toastmasters, or any other Talking group.

Do you think that open-minded communication is your best test? Join a formal club such as Toastmasters which will give you a stable method and opportunities to overcome this challenge. Furthermore, it's a fantastic way to make new acquaintances.

6. Practice by saying yes

Try to say"yes" to all invitations within the specified time period (multi-month is a good measure). By limiting yourself to different situations and situations, you'll force yourself to exercise your extrovert tendencies.

7. Take a moment to let yourself loose.

Do the thought of going to the upcoming Friday's vacation office gathering put you into the mood for a frenzied party? Allow yourself to go by focusing on a period of approximately 45 minutes of attendees, then after that it's "permitted" to leave. It's possible that you'll appreciate being able to stay once you're there, or not, you'll realize that you're able to handle everything for the duration of 45 minutes. This can allow you to change your thoughts to recognize when it's time to go to the gym.

8. The strength of Parity fluid is impressively

If you take a sip every moment, do not become too dependent on your fluids--but be aware that it's a benefit in the event that it can help you. A few drinks (max) may help in the most stressful of circumstances, but it shouldn't be your first choice.

9. Find out where you are standing

In a systems management or gathering scenario are you inclined to embrace the dividers or head to the refreshment area and stay there? Think about the extroverts that you have met: None are likely to be seen stationary or in front of dividers. Instead, make yourself visible in the room and listen to engage in conversations.

When you're in front of an individual, gaze at them straight on and keep a distance of about 2 feet. Make sure you stand in a straight line with the person you're talking to and also. This will help you in building a more personal connection with them.

10. Imagine you're playing host

When a wedding is being held, those who have newly pledged focus on going to each table, interacting with every person, and not focusing onto only those they trust. Imagine that you are the host at every occasion you attend, and engage with as many of guests you can.

You'll be expected to do this in situations of business as well as at events for systems administration. The practice makes perfect.

11. Concentrate on the task with total attention.

The most captivating people are usually the most effective audience members. This is where introverts are able to surpass expectations because they're skilled at being a good audience member. Be curious, ask to follow-up with questions, and demonstrate genuine passion for what other people are saying. It's not just your normal routine and it can cause you to appear attractive.

12. Keep up-to-date with the latest news

If you're planning to make an effort to attend an event you're attending, make sure to create a fast list of Google's most popular news articles (or any other media outlet you like). This will aid you in staying up-to-date on the latest news and also allow you to talk with anyone. Every pioneer must establish a system of skills that they normally do not have. Learning about the latest news can assist in solving problems in the absence of collaboration with the other person with whom you're communicating with.

13. Locate the icebreakers in the room

Whatever it is, whether it's an individual's fascinating adornments or the most unique thing in a quiet store take a few items that can be used to break the ice and make use of them to further enhance your advantages. This can be done in a professional setting or at a casual bar.

14. Stay off your cell phone

This could be a great test for extroverts and introverts alike. However, it is something you've seen before. In the event that it is it is possible, don't even take your phone with you. It's simply too appealing.

15. Do you have a few stories available

Everyone needs to have some good stories and jokes to pass around. If you're going to an industry conference, take a look at a few interesting news articles or tidbits that you can find interesting.

It's not easy to shift your lines, but it's doable. Practice prompts flawlessness, so remain over your extroversion amusement. It's hard to be shy in business However, the more you use these suggestions to your advantage, the better it'll benefit your company.

10 Things That Only Introverts with a personality who is outgoing would understand

Extrovert or introvert? You can think of it as a range in which you'll at some point in a time be on one side or the opposite. The majority of experts will be in the middle. They are referred to as Ambiverts. Outgoing introverts are definitely in this position, but people do not realize this and assume that they will be they are. Outgoing introverts know this extremely well. Here are ten things they'll be able to resonate with since life isn't always easy.

1. They believe that extroversion is overcompensated by the general public.

They might have participated in group projects at school, and collaboration, when used, but they believe that a quieter time to reflect and the ability to work with no one else should be more admired when working. It is not common for them to work in groups or in a team.

2. They could be the lifeblood and spirit of the gathering

Introverts who are outgoing can be lively entertaining, bubbly, and an excellent host at gatherings. They'll be exhausted within a few minutes and may not have any desire to be seen for more than a few hours or even days!

3. They can be amazing salespeople

It is believed that the extrovert is the best person to get the sale, however introverts who are outgoing have an abundance of options available to their career in sales it seems. They are aware of when to be quiet and when to push. They also excel at identifying a client's desires and needs.

4. They hate proms

Are you compelled to participate in certain events that can change your soul such as prom is an ideal way to get rid for some introverts who are outgoing. They'd prefer to be at home reading the book.

5. They are more likely to use social media

Social media has enabled many introverts with no social skills to adapt to each of the tricks that are dirty. It's social enough and allows for peace and quiet time with no interruptions. It's not necessary to go away from their normal range of familiarity. It's the perfect blend of engaging in social activities while remaining far from others!

6. They would rather be ignored at times

Sometimes, this causes irritation when they start to date. They may be friendly and great with friends, but then they might appear to fall back to themselves as they do not respond to messages or phone calls. The truth is their batteries in social life need renewal and that can't be done by themselves.

7. There isn't a lot of time to use phones.

One thing you can observe in these introverts is that they are extremely engaged, and don't have the ability to jump from one chatty post to an article or phone call. Talking and listening isn't a good idea with their deep thinking and focus.

8. They choose and select occasions to socialize

Going out can lead to lots of conversation which is totally worth it. They may appreciate social and group trips but you can bet that they'll be anxious when they are doing so. Other social occasions can be hazardous and dangerous for their safety. They could choose to follow the path of the least resistance or might appear to be to be pulled back.

9. They value introversion highly.

Stillness and moments of silence are generally viewed as negative. But, these qualities have led to some amazing discoveries and accelerated our progress as humans for quite a long time. The person who is outgoing regards their introversion as a high-quality one and has the perfect foundation to appear that way. They are extremely upset when people start to claim that something is wrong with their introversion!

10. They feel that it's difficult to change

There are issues when they have to go out regularly and perform like they are comics in a bazaar. They have in order to show their worth regarding, making friends or networks. They are aware of what society demands and wants. It's not always easy to turn on the extroversion of an electric light.

It's wonderful to be an introvert who is outgoing, but wouldn't it be great to have people understand them better?

Let us know in the comments about your experiences as an introvert who is outgoing can be a challenge or easy.

Normal Introvert Personality Characteristics

Introversion is among the most important personality traits that are that is a part of a myriad of theories about personality. Introverts tend to be internally focused or focusing more on their inner thoughts, feelings and attitudes, rather than seeking out external stimuli. In general, introversion is thought of as an aspect of a continuum that includes extraversion. Introversion is a signpost to one side of the spectrum, whereas extraversion demonstrates the opposite side.

Introverts tend to be more reserved, quiet and considerate. In contrast to extroverts who thrive through social interaction introverts must exhaust their their energy in social settings.

Basic Introversion Traits

Introversion is distinguished by a variety of sub-traits:

Extremely alert

Attentive

Apreciates the ability to comprehend subtle aspects

138

Inspiring with self-information, self-comprehension and the self

The tendency is to keep private feelings

Peaceful and kept in large groups or in new

More sociable and friendly when they are with friends and family members.

Well adapted by observing

How does introversion influence behavior?

What are the effects of introversion on how we behave? The most important thing to remember is that not all introverts are same. Some people are shy, while others are slightly or somewhere in between.

The ways that introversion could influence behavior include the following:

Introverts might have fewer and more close acquaintances. Researchers have observed that people who are high in this characteristic tend to live in a small circle of friends. Although extroverts for the majority have a large friends and colleagues network Introverts tend to select their acquaintances more carefully. The closest connections they have tend to be important and significant. They prefer to connect with each other on a personal basis rather than in an enormous group environment.

Success tips for introverts of all kinds

It's not always in all way easy, especially in an (western) world where extrovert individuals are more valued or in more precise terms they are in an superior position due to their personality which allows them to achieve their goals through many interactions and becoming more decisive with others and powerful chains of control. Many introverts could achieve significantly more on the possibility that they'd develop some social skills or put their energy in a particular skill usually attributed to extroverts in the form of a character attribute.

There are a number of advantages that come from being an introvert . These are qualities people who are introverts also often not aware of, for instance, that they aren't abusing their introverts. It's the time to come to an end to that.

Why are you an introvert?

Intriguing qualities of introverts and their misuse

Inexpensiveness of introverts and how to fix them

A few ways to be a successful introvert are having a switch that allows you to turn into an extrovert in an indefinite period of time, and focussing more on eminence rather instead of the strength

TRANSFROVERTED VERSUS EXTROVERTED PEOPLE

To be able to monitor, you should first understand it. Therefore, you should to first look at some bolts and nuts, and also the key distinctions between extroverts and introverts.

For instance, if recharge your energy batteries especially your mental and emotional ones, through social interaction it is likely that you're an extrovert. Likewise, if you recharge your energy sitting alone or in a peaceful setting, then you're probably an introverted type of person.

Introversion refers to the desire to focus on the inner world, pondering thoughts and seeking to understand extraversion refers to a preference for the external world, which includes objects, people and an urge to be active.

A shy person must be able to comprehend, while an extrovert person should behave. We can find the reason behind that in the first dimension. Experts have found that introverts are extremely sensitive to dopamine, the synapse which helps control the reward and pleasure centers - and that the part of the brain known as amygdala is extremely active with the connection (introverts have a an extremely delicate amygdala) Therefore, introverts may experience a rapid feeling of being overwhelmed.

In contrast, extroverts are an extremely low level of dopamine-related affect and thus require an extensive amount of external stimuli. The reason for this will be that the boosts travel in a more engrossing manner through the brains of introverts. Understanding which can aid you in understanding that introversion isn't only an individual characteristic, but an aspect of the sensory system.

Pay attention to one's inner movements of clairvoyance.

Appreciate solitude, perusing, exploring, reflecting

Harmony and calm are essential for focusing properly.

The best work is when you are only there.

Focus on deep one-on-one conversations and don't know how to have casual conversations.

They are usually surrounded by their family members and friends, and do not like large gatherings of people.

They may appear silent and reserved, however, they may have difficulty expressing.

Do You Want to Be an Extrovert or an Introvert?

The study suggests that extroversion may be can be linked to positive feelingswhich means that people who are more outgoing generally be happier than introverts. So, is this true? Psychotherapists who looked into this issue discovered that people who are extroverts typically feel more optimistic than introverts. In any event, scientists have also found evidence to prove that there are "cheerful introverts" When analysts looked at happy participants in the course of an examination, they discovered that 33% of them were also introverts. In other words, more extrovert people might experience positive emotions generally more frequently however, a lot of happy folks are also introverts.

Extrovert and Introvert are terms used by analysts for quite some time to define the character. As of late analysts have seen these traits as an important element of the five-factor show which is used to assess the personality. Analysers who analyze introversion and extroversion have realized that these distinctions have significant consequences for our happiness and behavior. In addition, research suggests that each method of being a part of a group has advantages and, at time, however, it's not feasible to claim that one method is superior to the other.

5 Personality Traits that Extroverts Display

Do you like being around new people? Are you a social event that can leaves you feeling inspired and rejuvenated? If you're able to answer "yes" to these questions, then it is possible that you might become an extrovert.

There's a lot of discussion these days about the distinction between introverts and extroverts, which is are often viewed as an either/or attribute. Introversion and extroversion are two of the primary personality indicators that comprise an overall model of five personality factors. Based on this assumption the personality is comprised of five thorough studies. Each measure, including extroversion/introversion, exists on a continuum. While some people might generally be on the extreme side of of the spectrum but the vast majority reside in the middle.

Even though you could have many traits that can make you an extrovert you might also find yourself having characters that seem more.

What is an Extrovert?

On the bright side, people who are extroverts are frequently depicted as cheerful, agreeable and organized in their activities, enthusiastic at ease, and open. On the other hand they can be are depicted as chasing attention quickly distracted, insufficient to focus on their own energy.

Some of the common characteristics of extroversion are:

Many, diverse interest

Likes to communicate through speech

Appreciates being at a focal factor of consideration

Will generally first act before examining

Appreciates work in general

Feels lonely due to an excessive amount of time spent by the loneliness of

Seeks out people around you and other hotspots on the outside for inspiration and inspiration

Loves to talk about thoughts and feelings

Extroverts have been linked to a variety of unique outcomes. One of the most beneficial results is that people who are extroverts generally have more fun in social interactions, invest more time engaged in activities that involve social interaction, and generally have more friends. The research has also indicated that extroverts generally be happier than introverts, and are less prone to a particular mental problems.

However, those who are extroverts are also likely to engage in risk taking practices, such as risky wellness behaviors.

You think you're an extrovert? Check out our list of five essential features that are essential to this kind of persona.

1.) You Love to Talk

You aren't content with just talking with family members, friends and colleagues You also enjoy striking off with a group of outsiders. You enjoy meeting strangers and learn the details of their life. In contrast to introverts who typically think before speaking extroverts will generally speak to help them investigate and clarify their thoughts and thoughts.

Extroverts, too, will generally have a large network of friends. Because you're so adept in making new acquaintances engaging in discussions, and you love the structure of other people, it likely won't come as a surprise that your creation partners are a success.

2.) Socializing makes you feel inspired and energized

Do you generally find yourself feeling "energized" and upbeat after spending some time with others? People who are extroverts generally experience social connections as enjoyable, and get more power from such exchanges. When people who are extroverts have to put in massive amounts of energy and are often left to feel tired and grumpy. When faced with the choice between spending their energy on only one thing and spending time with others the extrovert will often join an audience.

3.) You enjoy solving problems by discussing them

If you're faced with an issue, it is a good idea to discuss the issues and possible solutions with other people. Talking about it helps you look into the issue inside and out, and figure out what option is most effectively. After a stressful day at school or at work talking about it with your friends or with your family members will allow you to be less stressed. People who are introverts prefer to contemplate questions and focus on themselves after a difficult day.

4.) People have described you as friendly and approachable

Because those with this personality like to be around others so much they generally find them easy to talk to. When gatherings are held one can expect an extrovert to be the first to walk through the crowd and give presentations. Extroverts frequently think it's easy meeting new individuals and form new acquaintances.

5.) You're Very Open and Easy to Get to Know

Though introverts can be perceived as aloof and withdrawn typically, extroverts are welcoming and eager to share their opinions and thoughts. This is why other individuals, for greater of the time, feel that extroverts have less of a need to get to know each other.

Be aware that extroversion isn't a big or bust attribute It's a continuum and there are some who may be extremely extroverted whereas others aren't as. Extroversion is more prevalent than introversion, and is often considered a desirable trait since extroverts are generally have a knack for collaborating with other people. It doesn't necessarily mean, however that one type of personality is superior to other. Every type has its particular advantages and disadvantages and you might find that you're extroverted in some situations, and more introverted in other.

Chapter 9: Most Common Myths

If you think that you are an extrovert, you might have categorized an introvert as a 'party pooper'. You may find him in the corner in a quiet spot, watching the crowd like an eagle. You gave him a shot to speak with him and attempted to start some conversation. It was a mistake because the subject of conversation was so serious, it caused you to feel uncomfortable.

If you're an introvert, you might be feeling ostracized at one time and are unable to comprehend how a "party animal". It is difficult to comprehend why someone has the motivation to stay out late and get to know so numerous people. According to your experience it is that you go to the weekend party to dance, and enjoy several drinks with your buddies before leaving after feeling exhausted.

It doesn't matter if we like it or we don't the world is afflicted by stereotypes, and those with an introverted personalities are typically portrayed in a negative picture. Because introverts make up a small percentage with only 25 percent or 30 percent of population. It is true that the society of today has a an affinity for those that we believe to be extroverts-- people who are outgoing enthusiastic, confident and enthusiastic. Many of us believe that people who are bold are good people, and the more friends you make, the happier you'll be.

As children our parents want us to be less shy. We are encouraged to play outdoors with our friends or join clubs, and even participate in summer camps in order to build our social skills so that we can be successful in our lives. We are taught from a young age in life that the ideal self is one who enjoys being with the limelight. We view introversion as a second-class character trait, a failure or even a disease at its lowest. Parents continually urging their children to break out of their shells and often apologize to strangers for the awkwardness or shyness of their children.

The American Psychological Association's guidebook of mental disorders dubbed Diagnostic and Statistical Manual (DSM) could have been close to defining introversion to be a disorder of personality. (Interesting fact that homosexuality was classified as a disorder in the initial version of DSM). The positive thing about the current version of DSM (DSM-IV) It was accepted that social shyness is common and is not always an indicator of disease.

What led to this stigma against introverts as well as a an affinity for extroverts? We know that in the past there was a "Culture of Character' as cultural historian Warren Susman put it where we gave more importance to those with a calm and stoic manners. It was a time in which the economy was based on agriculture, and people lived side-by-side with people they knew for many years and all who lived in the same town.

Then came the second century, an era of large businesses, where people were lured to relocate to large cities and to interact with strangers. Naturally, the surroundings made people make themselves stand out, thereby promoting the "Culture of Personality'. People began to be attracted to the charismatic and friendly person. The man who is active was the preferred choice over the one who sat in contemplation. The modern world caused us to forget the ability of solitude, and we began to view introversion as a negative character trait.

Carl Jung developed introversion and extrovertivity for the purpose of describing the characteristics or attitudes of different individuals and not to categorize or create biases towards a particular kind of person. Here are some common assumptions we hold about introverts , and the reasons for why they are not true.

1. People who are introverts are not social.

It's an evocative word. If you search for it on the internet, antisocial could refer to an aggressive and dangerous behavior toward others. People who are introverts love being alone however it doesn't suggest that they are prone to hostile behavior.

This doesn't mean that introverts aren't averse to people. Actually introverts love to establish the trust of only one person at a. Many introverts enjoy with socializing, however they prefer to talk just when they've something meaningful to communicate. After a night out introverts need time to themselves to recharge.

2. Introverts aren't a fan of parties.

It might surprise you to find out that introverts like going out to clubs or bars but not for very long period of time. Their reason for going to a gathering is to be with their group of friends rather than in order to make new acquaintances. At large parties, introverts tend to watch the crowd instead of being the focus of attention.

3. People who are introverts are typically shy.

It is not the same as introversion. It is more about the fear that a person has of being judged. In contrast, introversion, as described in the beginning of chapter is the preferential choice for less stimulation. There are shy introverts. However, there are also extroverts that are shy.

4. The boring introverts.

Sitting at home by yourself or outside in the natural surroundings might appear boring, for certain people, but it is not the case for introverts. They feel content and happy in solitude, however, they also enjoy being with their family and close family. They don't want to engage in sports that provide adrenaline However, they engage with other activities outdoors as.

5. The introverts aren't allowed to speak in public.

Many introverts excel at public speaking. They would rather be in the presence of large audiences instead of introducing small talk sessions. According to what Jung said introverts are extremely intelligent and enjoy deep conversations. Talks of a small size are not appropriate for them as they can get the impression that they are not sincere. The sharing of an informative summary they created on a particular issue to a larger audience is more enjoyable for introverts.

In addition, introverts are excellent public speakers since they are prepared and practice more than extroverts.

6. People who aren't naturally inclined can't be leaders.

Our common sense would suggest that the most effective leaders are the most dominant and outgoing people in the crowd. What if we told you that transformative leaders such as Gandhi, Mother Theresa and Rosa Parks are introverts? They never wanted the spotlight however, they did made themselves known since every part of their bodies believed they were committed to a bigger cause.

Research studies have also shown that introverts are excellent listeners and encourage an exchange of thoughts within their teams. Introvert leaders are always looking at the bigger picture and are not be as likely to credit for the efforts of a skilled and active subordinate.

A study of Wharton faculty member Adam Grand found that introvert leaders have more outcomes. The reason is that introverts permit their employees to take charge of their own ideas. Extrovert leaders usually dictate how a particular project should be implemented and discourage proactive employees who may have the most innovative idea.

Introvert versus Extrovert

Extraversion, extrovert, or extraversion are not an opposite to introverts and introverts. Extrovert and introversion are component of one spectrum, or continuum. According to Jung, "no one is an absolute introvert or extrovert or extrovert, and they will end up in a mental institution". It is possible to be mostly extrovert or introvert however, nobody is at the edge of the range.

In order to help us recognize our predominant personality traits The following are the distinct physiological evidence and behavior manifestations of introverts and extroverts.

The Brain

In 1999, scientists employed in 1999, scientists used a PET scan to determine the flow of blood in the brains of introverts and extroverts when they were thinking freely. They discovered that there was an increase in the flow of blood in the frontal lobes, as well as the anterior thalamus areas in introverts. These brain regions play a role when it comes to memory, planning, and problem solving. Extroverts have more blood flow to the temporal lobes as well as the posterior thalamus regions which are involved in the interpretation of sensory inputs and the memory storage for new memories.

Researchers from the brain also observed the differences in dopamine levels of extroverts and introverts. Dopamine can be described as a neurotransmitter which transmits signals from the brain to the vital regions in our body. Dopamine influences our movements as well as our attention and emotional reactions. It has been reported the introverts possess higher amounts dopamine, making them more sensitive to stimuli. However the extroverts are less sensitive to stimuli. levels of dopamine. This makes them more prone to seeking stimulation from outside.

A 2012 research conducted by Harvard psychology professor Randy Buckner suggested that people who are mostly introverts tend to have greater amount of gray matter in certain areas of the prefrontal cortex. This is a brain region that is that is responsible for abstract reasoning and making decisions, whereas those who are classified as extroverts tend to have less gray matter in these same regions.

Intelligence and Giftedness

Although introversion is seen as a negative trait however, it is often connected with giftedness and intelligence. It is said that 70% of gifted individuals consider themselves introverts (e.g. Albert Einstein and Charles Darwin).

In addition introverts have been proven to have more knowledge about various topics. Psychologists Eric Rolfhus and Philip Ackerman conducted tests on 141 college students in 20 different areas ranging from physics to the arts, to statistics and astronomy. They discovered that introverts were more knowledgeable than extroverts in 19 subjects, likely because introverts spend more time studying than socializing.

The psychologist Adrian Furnham also avers that introverts score higher at school than extroverts.

Responding to External Stimulus

The sensitivity of introverts to external stimuli was proven by a study carried out by Harvard professor Jerome Kegan. Kegan collected 500 four-month old babies and then exposed them to different stimuli, like a balloon popping, or the aroma of ruby alcohol. He found the fact that 20% of the infants react to these stimuli by crying, while the other did nothing. Kegan interviewed the subject in the following years and found that the majority the children who responded to the triggers grew to be introverts.

Another intriguing experiment was conducted during 2012 with the psychologist Russell Green. Green provided math-related problems for people who are introverted and extroverts to work on. Green provided varying levels of background noise as the participants were solving the questions. The results indicated that introverts did better with less background noise while the extroverts were more successful with more background noise.

Psychologist Elaine Erin explained in her article published in January 2012 published in Time Magazine that introverts have an insufficient threshold for external stimulation. They are energized by internal pursuits like studying or thinking. People who are introverts feel drained by external activities like socializing, while extroverts benefit their interactions and are energized even without it.

Risk-taking

Being sensitive to stimuli, introverts have a lower tendency be enticed by the world or from other people. They prefer to do the solitude of fishing, writing or reading since it provides them with the chance to concentrate on their own mental process. They also prefer to be attentive to every angle before entering the situation, making them risk-takers of a moderate or minimal level.

Extroverts are classified as risk-averse, and this applies to all areas of life. Because they continuously seek stimulation from outside to boost their energy levels, people who are extroverts are more likely to participate in high-risk sports as well as other things like gambling or sexual activity that is unsafe. Another study revealed that extroverts possess a more active reward system within their brains. They are overly excited and will likely "go in the direction of it" when they spot something they would like to have, like the prospect of promotion or a lucrative investment. They get too focused on the rewards that they forget the warning signs.

A study of a group of traders working in the London Investment bank demonstrated that introverts had higher success than traders who were extroverts. This could be due to their mindset towards risk taking. Another example is Warren Buffet who describes himself as an introvert. Buffet declared that it was not his expertise that helped him become an investment expert, but his character.

Work Style

Psychologists have discovered that introverts are slower and more determined in completing a range of tasks. They also tend to tackle them one at one at a time. They are also noted by their capacity to focus on any task at hand.

Extroverts can complete tasks in shorter amounts of time, and are known as multi-taskers.

Communication

Scientists have suggested that the different in brain activity of people who are introverts and extroverts could have something to do with their style of communicating.

Introverts are more comfortable listening than speaking and can express themselves better through writing. Extroverts are more comfortable talking than listening, and are often themselves lost in words, and would often utter a few sentences they did not intend to say.

Introverts also tend to be more specific when describing things and be more precise in their descriptions compared to extroverts who tend to be less detailed and tend to concentrate on their emotions when communicating.

The type of clothing you wear

Based on a study conducted of RS Sharma, introverts prefer sensible and comfortable clothes and accessories, while extroverts tend to wear more aesthetically pleasing clothes.

The levels of happiness

Extroverts are believed to have reported higher levels happiness than introverts. This has led to the belief that introverts suffer from periods of depression. This isn't the reality. It is emphasized that the need for solitude in introverts is not an indication of depression, but it is a requirement to get their energy back after exposure to our extremely extroverted society.

Although people who are more extroverts have been found to be more prone to happiness, researchers asked whether they truly feel happier or simply more open about their emotions.

Benefits of Introverts

The introverts have a disadvantage over extroverts by about three-to-one. They can be often misunderstood even by their family and their friends. It is now known that the modern world is in harmony with an extroverted society. People prefer the charismatic and'socially adapted one. In spite of all chances, introverts discover an opportunity to flourish because of the wonderful characteristics they possess that the majority of us think of as normal.

Here are a few things that give introverts a leg up in our highly extroverted culture.

1. Interrupters are not allowed to interrupt someone who is talking.

Have you heard the expression "less talks, more errors"?

Introverts are more likely to think about information first , rather than expressing opinions in a few places. If an introvert isn't talking this doesn't mean that it's because he's uninterested or indifferent. It is more likely that he is to be thinking about ideas and analyzing them which he could communicate when the moment is appropriate.

2. Introverts are neutral.

Also they do not judge. They'd rather examine the reasons why someone behaves in a particular way and analyze their own behavior. It is less likely for them to spread negative remarks as well as get involved in gossip.

3. Introverts are honest.

If introverts speak be sure to believe the words were carefully selected and said with sincerity. They don't argue or sugarcoat or get off-topic. Meetings are comfortable when the person they are meeting with is direct and honest straight and to the main point.

4. Introverts can be great friends.

If you are faced with an important decision, be sure that your introvert friend will be more than happy to serve as your advocate and help you understand the advantages and disadvantages of the things. People who are introverts prefer quality over quantity in friendship. If an introvert has selected to be a friend of yours and you've chosen to be a friend, it's likely that your friendship will be for the rest of your life.

5. Introverts' motivation stems from the inside.

They don't require people or things that are material to fuel them. They can recharge themselves and build strength in the solitude that helps them flourish and remain resilient through tough times.

6. Introverts are extremely imaginative.

While they are generally analytic, introverts also dedicate lots of time to their imaginations and imaginative thinking. It is evident that a large number of creative people produce their most creative work when they are spending the majority of their time in a peaceful space. Some examples of creative individuals who describe themselves as introverts are the likes of Dr. Seuss and J.K. Rowling.

7. Introverts have the ability to manage their thoughts and feelings.

Introverts are able to develop a self-awareness consequence of the duration they devote in contemplation. They can pinpoint the cause of an unhappiness or emotion , and then try to change it. There is a very rare chance to hear someone who is introverted crying or yelling in public.

Benefits of Introverts to the Corporate World

In the competitive business world introverts are often referred to as"the quiet storm". Many may believe that they lack a lot of engagement due to them being uninterested in large group meetings. If we examine the issue the introverts will end up being best contributors and indispensable participants in the group.

They might not put a lot of emphasis on networking but you can trust them to remain in a calm, focused manner when the pressure is on. They are said to be superior in managing complex projects. procedures. These characteristics at work are the main reason they are the preferred choice for managers to hire because they have found introverts to be reliable and accountable.

They are also regarded as competent negotiators as they don't force their own ideas down someone or someone else's throat. Negotiation is done by speaking calmly and with a sense of humour asking questions and taking notes on the answers, which helps build trust and rapport.

They are also good leaders and mentors. The leaders who belong to the introvert group are interested in the larger cause than feeding one's own self-interest. Communications studies instructor Preston Ni coined a term she called soft power. As per Ni, "if your idea is sound and you act by the heart of your being, then it's an unwritten law that you'll draw people who are eager to support your cause. Soft power is the quiet persistence."

The advantages of introverts on the Dating World

Studies have proven that introverts have the ability to form lasting relationships more than extroverts. This is due to introverts being good listeners and can make their loved ones feel truly valued. Introverts also aren't shy about discussing more serious topics that can lead to an atmosphere of intimacy within the relationship. Discussions about serious subjects do not mean that there is drama. For introverts, speaking your inner thoughts and emotions is more appealing over casual conversations. The biggest advantage for introverts when it comes to dating is their capacity to make amends for their own mistakes. Due to their reflective nature introverts tend to apologize when they realise the actions of their partner caused them to be upset, and are likely avoid repeating the same error again.

Dealing with Extroverted Society

Perhaps you've discovered if you're more of an extrovert or introvert. We're not affirming you should be an introvert. It is just that it's less desirable over being an extrovert, or in the opposite direction. If you are aware of and appreciate your personality congratulations.

If you think you're an introvert it's unfortunate that you have to appear more extrovert than you are, and to do things that take you away on a regular day basis.

Here are some helpful tips to help you cope with the extrovert culture we live in.

1. Learn to decline invitations if you do not want to go.

A few introverts try to portray themselves as extroverts due the pressures of life that can cause them to become exhausted. In addition, you could be lost when you constantly fight the person you really are. It's time to not feel shamed when you don't say yes to your loved ones. This will allow you to have more time to reflect and help you regain your energy.

For instance, Charles Darwin, who was reported to have turned down a number of dinner invitations, and spent much of his time on his own through the forest. (We do not mean that you must be the hermit.)

To prevent internal debates about when it comes to whether or not go You can establish an amount limit on the number of social events you go to at least once a week, or up to four times in a month. Any invitations that exceed your amount will result in an automatic no.

2. Find a quiet place at work or in school in which you are able to be completely alone.

Take a look at how classrooms and offices are constructed. You'll be able to see that there are plenty of spaces open to the public that have been specifically designed to foster interaction. Many projects are also completed in groups. Teachers and managers are of the notion that the most effective works were created through collaboration. This could be a problem for introverts as the solitude of their lives is essential to their creativity. Being able to spend time to yourself during the day can assist an introvert to deal with the overwhelming stimuli of the world.

3. Request a part of the group project you can complete on your own.

A group effort does not require that your coworkers must work all working together to complete every task on the list. Pick the part of the task you believe does not require the involvement of the entire team. Then inquire with the manager of your project if it is possible to complete it on your own. However, this doesn't mean you're free to walk away from the team once your task is complete. Keep working with your team may require your inputs and ideas.

4. Find someone with whom you can exchange thoughts with.

It's not necessarily a love affair Maybe you have a fellow introvert in your family or group of friends that will understand your thought process. Being an introvert might cause you to feel lonely particularly if you don't have the opportunity to share your thoughts and insights.

5. Your loved ones should be aware of the need to be alone.

Our family and friends who are highly extrovert do not have the ability to read minds. If you are locked in your room for an extended duration, they'll likely assume that you have problems or is down about something. Simply telling them you're tired and require to take a break will help avoid incorrect assumptions. It is also a good idea to inform them about introversion as well as the extroversion. They might also discover aspects of their own personality.

Highly successful introverts

The most innovative and successful individuals tend to question the status quo and push the limits. They excel in collaborating and pushing ideas. It is easy to believe that the most groundbreaking ideas are developed by people who are extroverts and collaborate constantly However, psychology researchers Gregory Feist and Mihaly Csikszentmihalyi looked into the lives of a few of the most innovative individuals, they discovered that they have an introverted personalities. They would say that their solitude is the key ingredient that has fueled their creative abilities.

We've already mentioned some of the most famous introverts' names in the earlier chapters of the book however, there are many more that we'd like to discuss with you.

1. Albert Einstein

Einstein is quoted as in saying "The silence and monotony of a life that is quiet inspires creativity." Einstein once also stated, "When I examine myself and my thought processes I come to an understanding that my power of fantasy has been more meaningful in my life than any ability in abstract positively thinking."

2. Rosa Parks

The revolutionary leader who defeated racism in the 1950s was described with a lot of care by the author Susan Cain, "I had always thought of Rosa Parks as a stately woman with a strong personality and the ability to face a swarm of disgruntled passengers. However, when she passed away in 2005, at the age of 92 The flood of obituaries described her as soft-spoken sweetand diminutive in size. People said she was shy and shy, but she had the strength of an leopard. They used phrases such as radical humility and calm courage."

3. Bill Gates

On one interview, Gates answered a member of the audience who wanted to know how he was able to be successful in an extrovert environment "Well I think introverts are able to do pretty well. If you're smart and have the right mindset, you can gain the advantages of being an introvert. This could include, for instance, the ability to shut down for a couple of days to explore a challenging issue and read as much as you can, and push yourself to think in the zone. When you've have an idea that you would like to recruit people, get them excited, and build an organization around it You must learn about the ways that extroverts work, and you should hire extroverts like Steve Ballmer I would claim as an extrovert. You can utilize the strengths of both to build an enterprise that is successful both in the realm of deep thinking as well as creating teams and then taking the idea to the world to promote the ideas."

4. Warren Buffet

Buffett is averse to public speaking whenever he can and is based in Omaha away from the frantic world associated with Wall Street. He was quoted as saying "Once you've got a normal intelligence What you require is the ability to manage the desires that can lead investors in trouble"

Writer Susan Cain described Buffets introvert attributes, "intellectual persistence, prudent thinking, and the capacity to recognize and respond to warning signs to make hundreds of millions for him and his shareholders of Berkshire Hathaway, his business. Berkshire Hathaway"

5. Steve Wozniak

If you don't already know about Steve Wozniak, Steve Wozniak is the co-founder of Apple Inc. He created the first Apple computer while employed at Hewlett-Packard. He developed the initial design in his cubicle at HP and said he could not have become an expert had it not been for his introversion. He stated, "Most inventors and engineers I've encountered are just like me. They're shy and dwell in their heads. The most talented are artists. Artists work best on their own. They are not part of an organization. I am not on an individual team."

6. Theodor Geisel

The most well-known of them all is Dr. Seuss, he invented a lot of his fantastic characters inside the private bell tower that was used as his office on the rear of his home situated in La Jolla California. He claimed that meeting his readers, mostly children, can be a bit scary as they may be disappointed to learn that he isn't the jovial or energetic personality like the majority people he designed.

7. J.K. Rowling

Rowling said she was "quite an introvert" as did Her character Hermione. She said,

"Hermione is the character who is the one that is inspired by the real life person, and this person is me."

The writer also wrote "I wrote almost all the time since I was six years old, but I'd never been as enthusiastic about an idea before. My utter dismay, I did not have a pen that worked, and was too timid to ask anyone if they could get the pen... It was true that I didn't have a working pen However, I believe that it could have been an advantage. I just sat there and thought for about four (delayed train) hours, as the entire story exploded in my mind and this scrawny bespectacled black-haired man who had no idea that he was a wizard grew ever more real to me."

8. George Stephanopoulos

Journalist and advisor to the political Stephanopoulos has said in an interview in a newspaper, "Despite my job chatting people around I'm an introvert. It's been life-saving for me. I've been practicing meditation for around two years, regularly and a bit very seriously."

It's also a bit surprising that so many famous singers and actors are self-declared introverts. One would expect that these public figures are always seeking spotlights and company, however only they are not. A few of them have a place in the world of entertainment.

1. Audrey Hepburn

Hepburn openly admitted "I'm an introvert. I enjoy being alone and enjoy being outside. I take long walks with my dog and gazing at the flowers, trees and skies."

2. Angelina Jolie

Jolie has said, "I don't have a number of friends. I've been a bit lonely. What do you think? If you're by yourself If you travel somewhere and you're alone You end up meeting new people and develop."

3. Emma Watson

Watson quoted, "It's interesting, because people will say to me things like, 'It's awesome to not go out and drink every night and party that you can't go to.' I'm thinking, 'I know I'm grateful for that however, I'm an introverted type of person because of my nature. It's not something that I'm making. It's who I am,"

4. Keanu Reeves

As of 2005 Time magazine named Keanu Reeves as the world's most famous introvert. In an interview, he said, "I was kinda shy at school, however I had a character of a class clown. I was not a part of the class but I was also involved."

5. Courtney Cox

Cox declared, "I'm a homebody. I enjoy having friends over, but I'm bit unsocial. I'm not thrilled with it." She also blamed her divorce to personality differences "David loves to go to dance and go out. He's a social and sociable person. He's very social. I'm less of an introvert."

6. Christina Aguilera

Gabby Wood, a writer in Marie Claire magazine wrote about Aguilera, "She tells me that she's always been "intense and introverted and that is why she's felt as if she was an outsider all of her life."

Additional Interesting Facts About Introversion and Extroversion

We have already talked about introversion and extrovert as types of personality for humans. Would you believe that there are both types of personality all over our animal world? It's true! It is true that there are studies done by biologists regarding the introversion and extrovert of over a hundred species. Similar to the stats of humans, between 5 and 20 percent of all species have been described by biologists "sitters" or people who are seated on the sidelines and watch. The remaining 80 percent of them are "rovers" who move about and pay no at all to the environment around them. Let us present to you an experiment on people who sit and rove.